PET-CT-MRI-Based Cardiovascular Imaging

Editors

POUL FLEMMING HØILUND-CARLSEN
ABASS ALAVI
MATEEN C. MOGHBEL
ALI SALAVATI

PET CLINICS

www.pet.theclinics.com

Consulting Editor
ABASS ALAVI

April 2019 • Volume 14 • Number 2

ELSEVIER

1600 John F. Kennedy Boulevard • Suite 1800 • Philadelphia, Pennsylvania, 19103-2899

http://www.pet.theclinics.com

PET CLINICS Volume 14, Number 2
April 2019 ISSN 1556-8598, ISBN-13: 978-0-323-67841-4

Editor: John Vassallo (j.vassallo@elsevier.com)
Developmental Editor: Casey Potter

PET Clinics (ISSN 1556-8598) is published quarterly by Elsevier Inc., 360 Park Avenue South, New York, NY 10010-1710. Months of issue are January, April, July, and October. Periodicals postage paid at New York, NY, and additional mailing offices. Subscription prices per year are $240.00 (US individuals), $396.00 (US institutions), $100.00 (US students), $279.00 (Canadian individuals), $446.00 (Canadian institutions), $140.00 (Canadian students), $275.00 (foreign individuals), $446.00 (foreign institutions), and $140.00 (foreign students). To receive student and resident rate, orders must be accompanied by name of affiliated institution, date of term, and the signature of program/residency coordinator on institution letterhead. Orders will be billed at individual rate until proof of status is received. Foreign air speed delivery is included in all Clinics subscription prices. All prices are subject to change without notice. POSTMASTER: Send address changes to PET Clinics, Elsevier Health Sciences Division, Subscription Customer Service, 3251 Riverport Lane, Maryland Heights, MO 63043. **Customer Service: 1-800-654-2452 (U.S. and Canada); 314-447-8871 (outside U.S. and Canada). Fax: 314-447-8029. E-mail: journalscustomerservice-usa@elsevier.com (for print support); journalsonlinesupport-usa@elsevier.com (for online support).**

Reprints. For copies of 100 or more of articles in this publication, please contact the Commercial Reprints Department, Elsevier Inc., 360 Park Avenue South, New York, NY 10010-1710. Tel.: 212-633-3874; Fax: 212-633-3820; E-mail: reprints@elsevier.com.

PET Clinics is covered in MEDLINE/PubMed (Index Medicus).

Contributors

CONSULTING EDITOR

ABASS ALAVI, MD, MD (Hon), PhD (Hon), DSc (Hon)
Professor of Radiology and Neurology, Department of Radiology, Division of Nuclear Medicine, Hospital of the University of Pennsylvania, University of Pennsylvania Perelman School of Medicine, Philadelphia, Pennsylvania, USA

EDITORS

POUL FLEMMING HØILUND-CARLSEN, MD, DMSc, Prof (Hon)
Professor, Department of Nuclear Medicine, Odense University Hospital and Department of Clinical Research, University of Southern Denmark, Odense, Denmark

ABASS ALAVI, MD, MD (Hon), PhD (Hon), DSc (Hon)
Professor of Radiology and Neurology, Department of Radiology, Division of Nuclear Medicine, Hospital of the University of Pennsylvania, University of Pennsylvania Perelman School of Medicine, Philadelphia, Pennsylvania, USA

MATEEN C. MOGHBEL, MD
Department of Radiology, Stanford University Medical Center, Stanford University School of Medicine, Stanford, California, USA

ALI SALAVATI, MD, MPH
Department of Radiology, University of Minnesota, Minneapolis, Minnesota, USA

AUTHORS

ABASS ALAVI, MD, MD (Hon), PhD (Hon), DSc (Hon)
Professor of Radiology and Neurology, Department of Radiology, Division of Nuclear Medicine, Hospital of the University of Pennsylvania, University of Pennsylvania Perelman School of Medicine, Philadelphia, Pennsylvania, USA

RAMI AL-HADDAD
Department of Biochemistry, Microbiology and Immunology, University of Ottawa, University of Ottawa Heart Institute, Ottawa, Ontario, Canada

JOHN P. BOIS, MD
Department of Cardiovascular Diseases, Mayo Clinic, Rochester, Minnesota, USA

SIMON A. CASTRO, MD
Cardiac Electrophysiology, Cardiovascular Medicine Division, Hospital of the University of Pennsylvania, Philadelphia, Pennsylvania, USA

PANITHAYA CHAREONTHAITAWEE, MD
Department of Cardiovascular Diseases, Mayo Clinic, Rochester, Minnesota, USA

KEVIN CHEN, MD
Section of Cardiovascular Medicine, Yale School of Medicine, New Haven, Connecticut, USA

RAPHAEL ABEGÃO DE CAMARGO, MD, PhD
Specialist, Nuclear Medicine and Infectious Diseases, Postdoctoral Researcher University of Sao Paulo Medical School (FMUSP), Sao Paulo, Sao Paulo, Brazil; Nuclear Medicine Physician of Hospital São Rafael Rede D'Or, Hospital da Bahia, Clínica Diagnoson a+ Grupo Fleury and Hospital Aristides Maltez, Brazil

OKE GERKE, MSc, PhD
Chief Consultant, Biostatistician, Department of Nuclear Medicine, Odense University Hospital, Odense, Denmark

POUL FLEMMING HØILUND-CARLSEN, MD, DMSc, Prof (Hon)
Professor, Department of Nuclear Medicine, Odense University Hospital and Department of Clinical Research, University of Southern Denmark, Odense, Denmark

UZAIR S. ISMAILANI
Department of Biochemistry, Microbiology and Immunology, University of Ottawa, University of Ottawa Heart Institute, Ottawa, Ontario, Canada

SAURABH JHA, MBBS, MRCS, MS
Associate Professor of Radiology, University of Pennsylvania, Philadelphia, Pennsylvania, USA

JOEL S. KARP, PhD
Professor of Radiologic Physics, Chief of the Physics and Instrumentation Research Group, Department of Radiology, University of Pennsylvania, Philadelphia, Pennsylvania, USA

JACEK KWIECINSKI, MD
Cedars-Sinai Medical Center, Los Angeles, California, USA; British Heart Foundation Centre for Cardiovascular Science, University of Edinburgh, Edinburgh, United Kingdom

MARTIN LYNGBY LASSEN, PhD
Cedars-Sinai Medical Center, Los Angeles, California, USA

BEVERLEY CHERIE MILLAR, PhD
Clinical Scientist, Clinical Microbiology, Northern Ireland Public Health Laboratory, Department of Bacteriology, Belfast City Hospital, Belfast, Co. Antrim, Northern Ireland, United Kingdom

EDWARD J. MILLER, MD, PhD
Section of Cardiovascular Medicine, Yale School of Medicine, New Haven, Connecticut, USA

MATEEN MOGHBEL, MD
Department of Radiology, Stanford University Medical Center, Stanford University School of Medicine, Stanford, California, USA

JOHN EDMUND MOORE, PhD
Clinical Microbiologist, Northern Ireland Public Health Laboratory, Department of Bacteriology, Belfast City Hospital, Belfast, Co. Antrim, Northern Ireland, United Kingdom

DANIELE MUSER, MD
Cardiac Electrophysiology, Cardiovascular Medicine Division, Hospital of the University of Pennsylvania, Philadelphia, Pennsylvania, USA

CHRISTOPH RISCHPLER, MD
Department of Nuclear Medicine, University Hospital Essen, University of Duisburg-Essen, Essen, Germany

BENJAMIN H. ROTSTEIN, PhD
Department of Biochemistry, Microbiology and Immunology, University of Ottawa, University of Ottawa Heart Institute, Ottawa, Ontario, Canada

MEHRAN M. SADEGHI, MD
Section of Cardiovascular Medicine, Yale School of Medicine, New Haven, Connecticut, USA; Veterans Affairs Connecticut Healthcare System, West Haven, Connecticut, USA

PASQUALE SANTANGELI, MD, PhD
Assistant Professor of Medicine, Cardiac Electrophysiology, Cardiovascular Medicine Division, Hospital of the University of Pennsylvania, Philadelphia, Pennsylvania, USA

JEFFREY P. SCHMALL, PhD
Research Associate, Department of Radiology, University of Pennsylvania, Philadelphia, Pennsylvania, USA

PIOTR J. SLOMKA, PhD
Cedars-Sinai Medical Center,
Los Angeles, California,
USA

PAMELA K. WOODARD, MD
Mallinckrodt Institute of Radiology,
Washington University School of Medicine,
St Louis, Missouri, USA

Contents

Coronary computed tomography (CT) is one of the most rigorously tested imaging modalities. The history of evidence of coronary CT reflects the hierarchical model of efficacy of diagnostic imaging proposed by Fryback and Thornbury. Coronary CT has gone through technological evolution from electron beam CT to helical CT to multidetector CT. As technology improved, it also had to meet higher bars for evidence from proof of concept to diagnostic accuracy to evidence that it improves outcomes compared with its competitors.

Cardiovascular molecular imaging has focused on assessing myocardial perfusion and ventricular ejection fraction. These modalities target late downstream effects of the atherosclerotic disease process; this calls for a change of focus toward methods that can detect early arterial wall changes before macrocalcifications become visible on computed tomography angiography and provide a better understanding of the disease process. We summarize current knowledge on PET in atherosclerosis and highlight pertinent questions relating to the early detection of atherosclerosis. The future of PET in atherosclerosis may be early individualized quantification of the arteriosclerotic disease burden rather than exploration of features of individual arterial plaques.

PET-based cardiac nuclear imaging plays a large role in the management of ischemic heart disease. Compared with conventional single-photon emission CT myocardial perfusion imaging, PET provides superior accuracy in diagnosis of coronary artery disease and, with the incorporation of myocardial blood flow and coronary flow reserve, adds value in assessing prognosis for established coronary and microvascular disease. This review describes these and other uses of PET in ischemic heart disease, including assessing myocardial viability in ischemic cardiomyopathy. Developments in novel PET flow tracers and molecular imaging tools to assess atherosclerotic plaque vulnerability, vascular calcification, and vascular remodeling also are described.

The increasing implementation of advanced cardiovascular imaging in the form of cardiac PET/CT has had a significant impact on the management of cardiac sarcoidosis, which continues to evolve. This review summarizes the role of PET/CT imaging in sarcoidosis with a specific focus on (1) indications, (2) patient preparation, (3) test performance, (4) study interpretation, (5) clinical relevance of findings, (6) comparison to alternative imaging modalities, and finally (7) introduction of areas of anticipated development and research.

PET/MR Imaging in Cardiovascular Imaging   233

Christoph Rischpler and Pamela K. Woodard

With the emergence of PET/MR imaging there have been some strides in replicating the cardiovascular imaging success of other hybrid imaging modalities such as PET/computed tomography (CT) and single-photon emission computed tomography/CT. Because of the combined molecular imaging capabilities of PET and high-spatial and high-contrast resolution of MR imaging, there remains the potential for increased diagnostic accuracy and development of novel applications. In this article, the authors review the most promising cardiac PET/MR imaging applications developed since the introduction of PET/MR imaging in 2010 and summarize the most recent technical developments.

The Potential Role of Total Body PET Imaging in Assessment of Atherosclerosis   245

Jeffrey P. Schmall, Joel S. Karp, and Abass Alavi

Recent advances in molecular imaging and PET instrumentation will be of great value in assessing atherosclerosis plaques and other cardiovascular disorders. Atherosclerosis is systemic and involves critical arteries. Total body PET imaging will allow assessment of disease throughout the body as well as therapeutic monitoring. Because of the high sensitivity of total body PET, delayed imaging can be performed hours after administering tracer compounds, resulting in higher contrast at the disease site. Global assessment of the plaque burden throughout the body will substantially improve our ability to quantify plaque activity in the course of the disease.

PET/Computed Tomography Evaluation of Infection of the Heart   251

Beverley Cherie Millar, Raphael Abegão de Camargo, Abass Alavi, and John Edmund Moore

The 2015 European Society of Cardiology guidelines for the management of infective endocarditis included 18F-fluorodeoxyglucose (18F-FDG) PET/computed tomography (CT) in the diagnostic work-up of prosthetic valve endocarditis. This article examines the literature from the last 3 years to highlight the additional role 18F-FDG-PET/CT can contribute to an accurate diagnosis of cardiac infections and associated infectious complications. The challenges and pitfalls associated with 18F-FDG-PET/CT in such clinical settings must be recognized and these are discussed along with the suggested protocols that may be incorporated in an attempt to address these issues.

Gating Approaches in Cardiac PET Imaging   271

Martin Lyngby Lassen, Jacek Kwiecinski, and Piotr J. Slomka

Cardiac PET provides high sensitivity and high negative predictive value in the diagnosis of coronary artery disease and cardiomyopathies. Cardiac, respiratory as well as bulk patient motion have detrimental effects on thoracic PET imaging, in particular on cardiovascular PET imaging where the motion can affect the PET images quantitatively as well as qualitatively. Gating can ameliorate the unfavorable impact of motion additionally enabling evaluation of left ventricular systolic function. In this article, the authors review the recent advances in gating approaches and highlight the advances in data-driven approaches, which hold promise in motion detection without the need for complex hardware setup.

Daniele Muser, Simon A. Castro, Abass Alavi, and Pasquale Santangeli

Ventricular arrhythmias (VAs) are a major cause of morbidity and mortality, especially in patients with structural heart disease. In the last decade, advanced imaging modalities, such as cardiac MR and nuclear imaging, have progressively demonstrated to play a central role in the diagnosis and management of patients presenting with VAs. PET is acquiring a growing role thanks to its capability to assess different pathophysiologic aspects of the arrhythmogenic substrate by evaluating abnormal myocardial perfusion, presence of inflammation, myocardial viability, and sympathetic innervation. This review describes the principles and main clinical applications of PET imaging in the setting of VAs.

Rami Al-Haddad, Uzair S. Ismailani, and Benjamin H. Rotstein

PET imaging is a continuously developing clinical tool for the imaging of different markers of cardiovascular diseases. In this article, some important PET tracers for several diseases affecting the heart and the vessels are highlighted; these include myocardial blood flow, atherosclerosis, fatty acid metabolism, and pathologies in the cardiac autonomic nervous system.

PET CLINICS

SERIES OF RELATED INTEREST

MRI Clinics of North America
Available at: MRI.theclinics.com
Neuroimaging Clinics of North America
Available at: Neuroimaging.theclinics.com
Radiologic Clinics of North America
Available at: Radiologic.theclinics.com

THE CLINICS ARE AVAILABLE ONLINE!
Access your subscription at:
www.theclinics.com

PROGRAM OBJECTIVE
The goal of the *PET Clinics* is to keep practicing radiologists and radiology residents up to date with current clinical practice in positron emission tomography by providing timely articles reviewing the state of the art in patient care.

TARGET AUDIENCE
Practicing radiologists, radiology residents, and other health care professionals who provide patient care utilizing radiologic findings.

LEARNING OBJECTIVES
Upon completion of this activity, participants will be able to:
1. Review the principles and clinical applications of PET imaging in Ventricular arrhythmias
2. Discuss the history of evidence of the efficacy of coronary CT.
3. Recognize recent advances made in molecular imaging along with PET instrumentation in assessing Atherosclerosis plaques, and potentially other Cardiovascular related disorders.

ACCREDITATION
The Elsevier Office of Continuing Medical Education (EOCME) is accredited by the Accreditation Council for Continuing Medical Education (ACCME) to provide continuing medical education for physicians.

The EOCME designates this enduring material for a maximum of 15 *AMA PRA Category 1 Credit*(s)™. Physicians should claim only the credit commensurate with the extent of their participation in the activity.

All other health care professionals requesting continuing education credit for this enduring material will be issued a certificate of participation.

DISCLOSURE OF CONFLICTS OF INTEREST
The EOCME assesses conflict of interest with its instructors, faculty, planners, and other individuals who are in a position to control the content of CME activities. All relevant conflicts of interest that are identified are thoroughly vetted by EOCME for fair balance, scientific objectivity, and patient care recommendations. EOCME is committed to providing its learners with CME activities that promote improvements or quality in healthcare and not a specific proprietary business or a commercial interest.

The planning committee, staff, authors and editors listed below have identified no financial relationships or relationships to products or devices they or their spouse/life partner have with commercial interest related to the content of this CME activity:

Abass Alavi, MD, MD(Hon), PhD(Hon), DSc(Hon); Rami Al-Haddad; John P. Bois, MD; Simon A. Castro, MD; Panithaya Chareonthaitawee, MD; Kevin Chen, MD; Raphael Abegão de Camargo, MD, PhD; Oke Gerke, MSc, PhD; Poul F. Høilund-Carlsen, DM, DMSc, Prof(Hon); Uzair S. Ismailani; Saurabh Jha, MBBS, MRCS, MS; Joel Karp, PhD; Alison Kemp; Jacek Kwiecinski, MD; Martin Lyngby Lassen, PhD; Beverley Cherie Millar, PhD; Mateen Moghbel, MD; John Edmund Moore, PhD; Daniele Muser, MD; Christoph Rischpler, MD; Benjamin H. Rotstein, PhD; Ali Salavati, MD, MPH; Pasquale Santangeli, MD, PhD; Jeffrey Schmall, PhD; Piotr J. Slomka, PhD; John Vassallo; Vignesh Viswanathan; Pamela K. Woodard, MD.

The planning committee, staff, authors and editors listed below have identified financial relationships or relationships to products or devices they or their spouse/life partner have with commercial interest related to the content of this CME activity:

Edward J. Miller, MD, PhD: *is a consultant/advisor for General Electric and is a consultant/advisor for and receives research support from Bracco Diagnostics Inc.*

Mehran M. Sadeghi, MD: *is a consultant/advisor for Bracco Diagnostics Inc.*

UNAPPROVED/OFF-LABEL USE DISCLOSURE
The EOCME requires CME faculty to disclose to the participants:
1. When products or procedures being discussed are off-label, unlabelled, experimental, and/or investigational (not US Food and Drug Administration [FDA] approved); and
2. Any limitations on the information presented, such as data that are preliminary or that represent ongoing research, interim analyses, and/or unsupported opinions. Faculty may discuss information about pharmaceutical agents that is outside of FDA-approved labelling. This information is intended solely for CME and is not intended to promote off-label use of these medications. If you have any questions, contact the medical affairs department of the manufacturer for the most recent prescribing information.

TO ENROLL
To enroll in the *PET Clinics* Continuing Medical Education program, call customer service at 1-800-654-2452 or sign up online at http://www.theclinics.com/home/cme. The CME program is available to subscribers for an additional annual fee of USD $235.

METHOD OF PARTICIPATION

In order to claim credit, participants must complete the following:

1. Complete enrolment as indicated above.
2. Read the activity.
3. Complete the CME Test and Evaluation. Participants must achieve a score of 70% on the test. All CME Tests and Evaluations must be completed online.

CME INQUIRIES/SPECIAL NEEDS

For all CME inquiries or special needs, please contact elsevierCME@elsevier.com

Preface

PET-CT-MR Imaging-Based Cardiovascular Imaging

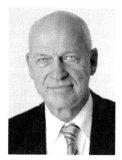
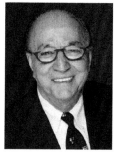
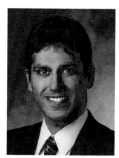
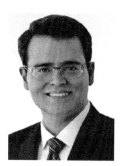

Poul Flemming Høilund-Carlsen, MD, DMSc, Prof (Hon)   Abass Alavi, MD, MD (Hon), PhD (Hon), DSc (Hon)   Mateen C. Moghbel, MD   Ali Salavati, MD, MPH

Editors

The past five decades have witnessed a major revolution in medical imaging, and this has had a profound impact on the management of many maladies, including cardiovascular disorders. Conventional planar x-ray imaging has been replaced by x-ray–based computed tomography (CT) for many medical indications. The introduction of MR imaging has further enhanced the role of structural imaging, particularly in the assessment of diseases and disorders that have affected the central nervous, musculoskeletal, and cardiovascular systems. In parallel with the advances that have been made in the detection of structural abnormalities visualized by CT and MR imaging, the evolution of functional and molecular imaging with PET has reshaped the role of medical imaging in many domains.

As the medical community started to utilize these powerful imaging techniques on a wide scale, it became clear that the sensitivity and specificity of structural imaging modalities are often suboptimal for the early detection of disease and the assessment of response to therapy. It is typically late in a disease process when changes on a physiologic level, such as blood flow and organ motility, lead to structural abnormalities that become apparent on modalities such as CT and MR imaging (**Fig. 1**). Therefore, relying on structural imaging for the management of many diseases can lead to delayed and often prolonged interventions and suboptimal outcomes. By contrast, molecular probes, which visualize pathology on a microscopic rather than macroscopic level, have the potential to detect disease and allow for intervention earlier in the process.

Cardiovascular imaging with radiotracer-based approaches has been primarily based on compounds that are labeled with single gamma emitters. While early applications of perfusion imaging techniques utilized planar data acquisition, over the past three decades such studies have been carried out by employing single-photon emission computed tomography (SPECT). Currently, SPECT perfusion imaging is the most commonly used imaging modality in the field of nuclear medicine for assessing atherosclerosis in the coronary arteries. However, SPECT imaging instruments suffer from poor spatial resolution and suboptimal quantification. Therefore, the sensitivity and specificity of this approach are somewhat limited, and as such, there is a dire need to introduce newer techniques with better performance.

During the past four decades, PET imaging with novel radiotracers has revolutionized the specialty of medical imaging. While initial applications of PET were confined to evaluating central nervous system disorders, with the introduction of advanced PET machines, it has become feasible to image every organ system in the body. Particularly, PET has become the imaging modality of choice in the management of a large number of

PET Clin 14 (2019) xiii–xv
https://doi.org/10.1016/j.cpet.2019.01.001
1556-8598/19/© 2019 Published by Elsevier Inc.

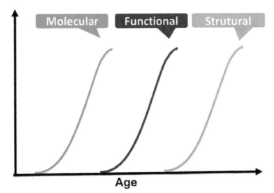

Fig. 1. The probable sequence of biological events as they relate to many disorders. Functional activities refer to physiological alterations, such as blood flow and organ motility. This pattern is particularly relevant to the assessment of atherosclerosis in the coronary arteries as well as other arteries. As such, molecular imaging with PET may provide early evidence of the disease process. (*From* Moghbel M, Al-Zaghal A, Werner TJ, et al. The role of PET in evaluating atherosclerosis: a critical review. Semin Nucl Med 2018;48(6):489; with permission.)

malignancies. To date, the workhorse for PET-based assessment of cancer has been ^{18}F-fluoro-deoxyglucose (FDG). However, widespread use of this technology has revealed its nonspecificity for cancer due to high uptake of FDG in inflammatory lesions. Attempts have been made to examine a variety of inflammatory disorders, including atherosclerotic plaques in the major arteries. However, the nonspecificity of FDG for detecting inflammation in the plaques has posed a significant challenge for visualizing and characterizing atherosclerosis in the arteries. Moreover, intense uptake of FDG in the myocardium has made it impossible to use this technique to detect inflammatory plaques in the coronary arteries. Therefore, other tracers have been introduced for assessing a variety of cardiovascular disorders, with an emphasis on atherosclerosis. Among these tracers, ^{18}F-labeled sodium fluoride (NaF) appears to be of particular promise for detecting molecular calcification in this degenerative process. This tracer is specific and also sensitive for the detection of molecular calcification in plaques at various stages of the disease. The preliminary data from many centers appear to be very promising, and as such, this approach may substantially improve our ability to assess patients with suspected or proven atherosclerosis and determine the impact of various interventions (**Fig. 2**). The role of other tracers that have been tested over the years is somewhat uncertain at this time due to the suboptimal spatial resolution of PET instruments in

detecting subtle pathologic changes in atherosclerotic lesions.

The introduction of PET-CT in 2001 has further enhanced the role of molecular imaging in the management of patients with cardiovascular disorders. X-ray–based CT has been extensively employed to detect structural calcification in the coronary and major arteries over the years. It is our view that structural calcification as noted on CT is of limited value since it reveals irreversible stages of the disease. When such abnormalities are visualized on CT scan, it is very likely that the disease process has been ongoing for decades and has therefore led to permanent damage. The data generated by adopting NaF-PET imaging suggest that this technique may become invaluable in the management of patients with coronary and other major artery atherosclerosis. In the past two decades, multislice CT has been employed to perform coronary arteriography with success. This methodology allows detection of vascular narrowing due to advanced atherosclerotic plaques. This has substantially eliminated the need for catheter-based arteriography, which was considered the gold standard prior to the introduction of cardiac CT. We believe the combination of PET with CT will substantially enhance the performance of both techniques in the detection and quantification of atherosclerotic lesions.

The introduction of MR imaging as a major imaging modality in the 1980s has further enhanced the role of imaging for examining cardiovascular disorders. MR imaging has been of great value in assessing soft tissue abnormalities in the cardiovascular system as well as in other organs in the

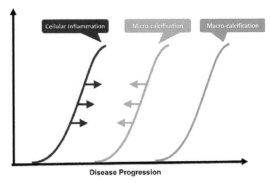

Fig. 2. The probable sequence of biological events in atherosclerosis. It is well known that endothelial inflammation and vascular microcalcification precede macrocalcification; thus, FDG and NaF PET could detect the earliest phases of the disease even in asymptomatic individuals. (*From* Moghbel M, Al-Zaghal A, Werner TJ, et al. The role of PET in evaluating atherosclerosis: a critical review. Seminin Nucl Med 2018;48(6):489; with permission.)

body. This is in contrast with CT imaging, which has been of limited value in this domain. Therefore, MR imaging for detecting cardiac and vascular abnormalities has played a major role in managing disorders that occur in the cardiovascular system. Claims have been made about the role of MR imaging in assessing disease processes on the molecular and cellular levels. Unfortunately, the limited sensitivity of this modality has impeded its success, and therefore, its impact as a molecular imaging probe with current instruments. However, PET-MR imaging as a combined modality will substantially enhance the role of each modality by visualizing and further characterizing abnormalities that are detected by PET.

Finally, the limited field of view of the current PET instruments has been an obstacle for optimal utilization of this technique in both clinical and research domains. In other words, the limited axial field of view requires 20 to 25 minutes of imaging within 1 to 2 hours following the administration of compounds such as FDG. High background activity in the vascular system during the first 2 hours adversely affects the sensitivity of this technique in detecting atherosclerotic plaques. Therefore, instruments that allow for imaging of the entire body simultaneously may further enhance the role of PET in examining cardiovascular disorders. In the past few years, attempts have been made to image the entire body with a substantially larger field of view and greatly enhanced sensitivity. The success of these efforts will strengthen the impact of PET imaging in this extremely prevalent disease. This approach allows for total body imaging in 3 to 5 minutes, 3 to 4 hours after the administration of molecular compounds, when the background activity has substantially decreased and is less of a barrier to accurate quantification of atherosclerotic burden.

In this issue of *PET Clinics*, we have included scientific communications that are currently of great interest to the medical community with regard to the performance of PET imaging techniques for both clinical and research applications.

Poul Flemming Høilund-Carlsen, MD, DMSc, Prof (Hon)
Department of Nuclear Medicine
Odense University Hospital and
Department of Clinical Research
University of Southern Denmark
Sønder Boulevard 29
Odense, 5000 Denmark

Abass Alavi, MD, MD (Hon), PhD (Hon), DSc (Hon)
Department of Radiology
Hospital of the University of Pennsylvania
3400 Spruce Street
Philadelphia, PA 19104, USA

Mateen C. Moghbel, MD
Department of Radiology
Stanford University School of Medicine
300 Pasteur Drive
Stanford, CA, 94305-5105, USA

Ali Salavati, MD, MPH
Department of Radiology
University of Minnesota
420 Delaware Street Southeast
Minneapolis, MN 55455, USA

E-mail addresses:
pfhc@rsyd.dk (P.F. Høilund-Carlsen)
Abass.Alavi@uphs.upenn.edu (A. Alavi)
mateenm@stanford.edu (M.C. Moghbel)
salavati@gmail.com (A. Salavati)

Coronary Computed Tomography: A Brief History

Saurabh Jha, MBBS, MRCS, MS

KEYWORDS

- Coronary CT • Diagnostic efficacy • Outcomes • Randomized controlled trials

KEY POINTS

- Coronary computed tomography (CT) is one of the most rigorously tested imaging modalities.
- Coronary CT is an incremental innovation.
- Coronary CT gate keeps catheter angiography.

INTRODUCTION

Shortly after the discovery of computed tomography (CT), researchers saw a role for CT in the evaluation of patients with suspected obstructive coronary artery disease (CAD). Specifically, role of CT would be to see the coronary arteries with roughly the same clarity as the diagnostic gold standard for CAD, catheter angiogram (CA). Coronary CT would serve 2 functions: diagnose CAD and save patients from unnecessary CAs.

Catheter angiography is an invasive test in which CAD is diagnosed planimetrically, that is, by measuring the degree to which plaque narrows the artery. Coronary CT would perform the same planimetric function as CA but with advantages, it would also see the plaque that does not narrow the artery but merely thickens the arterial wall, a phenomenon known as "positive vessel remodeling." Such plaque cannot be seen on CA because CA, a form of projectional imaging, is a luminogram, which sees the lumen of the artery, but not its wall. Coronary CT would save the patient from complications of catheter angiography, which are principally complications of arterial access.

The history of coronary CT is not merely the history of technological development of CT, but history of evidence. Coronary CT is one of the most rigorously tested imaging modalities. This article outlines the history of evidence of the efficacy of coronary CT.

EFFICACY OF TECHNOLOGY

In a landmark paper, Fryback and Thornbury[1] listed hierarchical goals that a new technology must fulfill as it diffuses. Technology must first prove technical feasibility, a proof of concept that it plausibly does what it sets out to do. Following technical efficacy, technology must prove diagnostic efficacy, that it has an acceptable accuracy for the disease it seeks, that is, sensitivity and specificity, when refereed by the gold standard of the disease. After diagnostic efficacy, technology must show therapeutic efficacy, that is, evidence that the information obtained from the imaging alters treatment decisions. Thereafter, imaging should show that the changed management, as a result of it, improves outcomes, meaning it adds quality-adjusted life-years. Finally, imaging should show that the improved outcome is a cost-effective use of finite societal resources.

Each stage in the diagnostic pyramid is necessary, although not sufficient, for the next step. For example, without technical efficacy, coronary CT cannot aspire toward diagnostic efficacy, and without diagnostic efficacy, it cannot achieve therapeutic efficacy.

Disclosure Statement: The author has nothing to disclose.
Hospital of University of Pennsylvania, 3400 Spruce Street, Philadelphia, PA 19104, USA
E-mail address: Saurabh.jha@uphs.upenn.edu

PET Clin 14 (2019) 193–195
https://doi.org/10.1016/j.cpet.2018.12.002

TECHNICAL AND DIAGNOSTIC EFFICACY OF CORONARY COMPUTED TOMOGRAPHY

The proof of concept that coronary arteries may be seen on CT was first supplied by electron beam computed tomography (EBCT). The technology, made obsolete by multidetector helical CT, had a high temporal resolution (shutter speed) because the tube did not have to be rotated mechanically. Instead, the focal point of the electron beam was moved electronically. Thus, EBCT was capable of high-temporal resolution and could see the moving coronary arteries.

The seminal study on coronary CT was published in the *New England Journal of Medicine* in 1998.[2] Researchers studied the technical efficacy and diagnostic performance of EBCT using CA as the gold standard. Researchers studied 125 patients who were going to have CA; thus, everyone received the gold standard. Only the proximal and midsegments of the coronary arteries were evaluated. Of the 500 coronary segments studied, 124 had to be excluded from analysis because of technical limitations. Nevertheless, EBCT identified 69 of the 75 segments with high-grade stenosis/occlusions and was correct in declaring in 282 of the 301 segments without high-grade stenosis, absence of CAD. Once the nonevaluable segments were excluded from the denominator, the researchers reported a respectable, albeit inflated, sensitivity of 92% and specificity of 94%.

Ironically, the evidence for the technological efficacy of magnetic resonance (MR) coronary angiography preceded CT by 5 years.[3] In that study, MR boasted a sensitivity of 90% and specificity of 92% for obstructive CAD. Nevertheless, CT marched ahead while MR was stuck in proof of concept. MRI's lag happened for three reasons happened for 3 reasons. First, although both improved technically, CT improved in 3 principal dimensions: acquisition time, temporal resolution, and spatial resolution. Spatial resolution, MR's Achilles heel, was CT's strength.

The principle drawback of EBCT was its low signal-to-noise: the images were noisy but EBCT still had a faster shutter speed than conventional CT around that time. With the discovery of the slip ring technology, CT could rotate and translate at the same time, that is, move and see. This movement is technically a helix. Thus, the new phenotype of CT became known as "helical CT," a term used interchangeably with "spiral." At the same time, vendors started packing CTs with detectors, and CT became multidetector computed tomography (MDCT). The 2 developments happened around the same time, and CT progressed in all fronts. Spatial resolution, contrast resolution, and temporal resolution improved contemporaneously, and CT became better at seeing small, moving structures, such as coronary arteries.

Ten years after EBCT displayed proof of concept, a study showed the diagnostic efficacy of MDCT.[4] The Coronary Evaluation using multidetector 64 CT (CorE 64) trial was a multicenter trial in which patients had CT before CA, just as they did in the trial involving EBCT. CT's performance was modest, but usable, with a sensitivity of 85% and specificity of 90%.

TOWARD OUTCOMES

An editorial accompanying the publication of the CorE 64 trial echoed the sentiments of Fryback and Thornbury that diagnostic efficacy was not enough for technology to be adopted.[5] Technology had to show that it improved outcomes, not merely that it successfully diagnosed the disease.

The gauntlet was thrown; coronary CT had 2 challenges. The first was that it had to show that it improved outcomes. The second was to show that it improved outcomes above and beyond the other tests. Coronary CT is no' the only modality for the detection of CAD. Alternative modalities include myocardial perfusion imaging (MPI), stress echo, PET, and exercise electrocardiogram.

The assessment of incremental benefits of competing technologies is known as comparative effectiveness. In the Prospective Multicenter Imaging Study for the Evaluation of Chest Pain (PROMISE) trial, patients with low-intermediate probability of chronic stable angina were randomized to either coronary CT (anatomic testing) or functional testing, such as MPI and stress echo.[6] The primary outcome, all-cause mortality, myocardial infarction, unstable angina hospitalization, or major complication from a cardiovascular procedure, occurred in 3.3% of the anatomic group and 3% of the functional group, but this small difference was not statistically significant. Patients randomized to anatomic testing were more likely to be catheterized than patients randomized to functional testing (12.1 vs 8.1%), but the positive yield of CAD on CA was higher for the anatomic group.

PROMISE showed that coronary CT was as good as its alternatives but not better. In the 5-year follow-up of the Scottish Computed Tomography of the Heart (SCOT Heart) trial,[7] researchers found that the rate of primary end point (death and nonfatal myocardial infarction) was lower in the group randomized to CT than the group randomized to functional testing (2.3% vs 3.9%). The rates of catheter angiography and revascularization were similar in both groups.

The difference appears to be driven by initiation and adherence to primary prevention, which was higher in the CT group (odds ratio 1.4). Thus, SCOT-Heart trial showed that CT did indeed improve outcomes, above and beyond its alternative modalities.

BEYOND ANATOMY

The test performance of CT is refereed by catheter angiography with the assumption that the gold standard, the truth, for obstructive CAD is planimetry, that is, greater than 50% stenosis in the left main and greater than 70% stenosis in the other epicardial coronary arteries. However, planimetry is a flawed gold standard, and a better, more hemodynamically representative, gold standard is fractional flow reserve (FFR) in which the hemodynamic significance of a stenosis is assessed by measuring the pressure drop across a stenosis during catheter angiography. FFR less than 0.8 is considered significant. The Fractional Flow Reserve versus Angiography for Guiding Percutaneous Coronary Intervention trial showed that therapeutic decisions based on FFR led to better outcomes than therapeutic decisions based on planimetry.[8]

Accordingly, vendors sought to determine FFR on CT; thus, again, obviating catheter angiography. FFR on CT is measured by complex flow models, that is, it is a simulation. FFR-CT is at the same place that coronary CT was during 2008: it is showing technical and diagnostic accuracy.[9] Sensitivity and specificity of FFR-CT is 90% and 54%, respectively. Thus, FFR-CT has some way to go before routine adoption.

FUTURE OF CORONARY COMPUTED TOMOGRAPHY

The plethora of options in imaging patients with chronic stable angina has taken the wind out of coronary CT. Nevertheless, the modality is useful because of its high negative predictive value and its ability to see plaque, both calcified and noncalcified. The prognostic information from CT is powerful and can be used to tailor preventive treatment. As the radiation doses continue to decrease, the case for using coronary CT as the first-line test to exclude obstructive CAD will become stronger.

REFERENCES

1. Fryback DG, Thornbury JR. The efficacy of diagnostic imaging. Med Decis Making 1991;11(2):88–94.
2. Achenbach A, Moshage W, Ropers D, et al. Value of electron-beam computed tomography for the noninvasive detection of high-grade coronary-artery stenosis and occlusions. N Engl J Med 1998;339:1964–71.
3. Manning WJ, Lei W, Edelman RR. A preliminary report comparing magnetic resonance angiography with conventional angiography. N Engl J Med 1993;328:828–32.
4. Miller JM, Rochitte CE, Dewey M, et al. Diagnostic performance of coronary angiography by 64-row CT. N Engl J Med 2008;359:2324–36.
5. Redberg RF, Walsh J. Pay now, benefits may follow – the case of cardiac computed tomographic angiography. N Engl J Med 2008;359:2309–11.
6. Douglas PS, Hoffmann U, Patel MR, et al. Outcomes of anatomical versus functional testing for coronary artery disease. N Engl J Med 2015;372:1291–300.
7. The SCOT-HEART Investigators, Newby DE, Adamson PD, Berry C, et al. Coronary CT angiography and 5-year risk of myocardial infarction. N Engl J Med 2018;379:924–33.
8. De Bruyne B, Pijls NHJ, Kalesan B, et al. Fractional flow reserve-guided PCI versus medical therapy in stable coronary artery disease. N Engl J Med 2012;367:991–1001.
9. Min JK, Leipsic J, Pencina MJ, et al. Diagnostic accuracy of fractional flow reserve from anatomic CT angiography. JAMA 2012;308(12):1237–45.

Evolving Role of PET in Detecting and Characterizing Atherosclerosis

Poul Flemming Høilund-Carlsen, MD, DMSc[a,b,*],
Mateen C. Moghbel, MD[c], Oke Gerke, MSc, PhD[a],
Abass Alavi, MD, MD (Hon), PhD (Hon), DSc (Hon)[d]

KEYWORDS

- PET/CT • PET/MRI • Atherosclerosis • Cardiovascular disease • FDG • NaF • Inflammation
- Calcification

KEY POINTS

- The use of ^{18}F-fluorodeoxyglucose and ^{18}F-sodium fluoride signifies a shift in focus of molecular imaging in cardiovascular disease, from imaging of late downstream effects of atherosclerosis to detection and characterization of active atherosclerosis in its early stages.
- Arterial wall inflammation and microcalcification are dynamic processes that are not directly interconnected.
- The frequency of arterial wall inflammation and microcalcification increases slightly with age, but only microcalcification correlates consistently with 10-year Framingham risk scores.
- The mainstay of PET imaging in atherosclerosis may shift toward early ^{18}F-sodium fluoride PET grading of atherosclerotic disease burden, rather than characterizing features of single plaques.
- ^{18}F-sodium fluoride PET imaging offers an individualized measurement of microcalcification in the heart, the aorta, carotids and other major arteries with a reproducibility allowing for monitoring of antiatherosclerotic interventions.

INTRODUCTION

Strategic PET imaging with ^{18}F-fluorodeoxyglucose (FDG) and/or ^{18}F-sodium fluoride (NaF) heralds a new era of molecular cardiovascular imaging. It will expand our understanding of atherosclerosis and allow us to shift our focus from the late to the early stages of atherosclerotic disease. If present promises hold true, it may even minimize or obviate most of the current actions we take against the disease.

Molecular imaging of cardiovascular disease (CVD) has been a success story from its beginnings in 1925, when Hermann Blumgart and Otto Yens used a modified Wilson cloud chamber to "image" the effects of α and β particles for the purpose of measuring delayed circulatory transit times in heart patients compared with normal controls.[1,2] The imaging milestones that followed included the visualization of the pulmonary circulation in the 1960s by George Taplin and by Henry

This article was not funded. The authors have nothing to disclose.
[a] Department of Nuclear Medicine, Odense University Hospital, J. B. Winsløws Vej 4, 5000 Odense C, Denmark; [b] Department of Clinical Research, University of Southern Denmark, Winsløwparken 19, 3. salOdense C - DK-5000, Denmark; [c] Department of Radiology, Stanford University Medical Center, Stanford University School of Medicine, 300 Pasteur Drive, Stanford, CA 94305-5105, USA; [d] Department of Radiology, Hospital of University of Pennsylvania, 3400 Spruce Street, Philadelphia, PA 19104, USA
* Corresponding author. Department of Nuclear Medicine, Odense University Hospital and Institute of Clinical Research, University of Southern Denmark, Sdr. Boulevard 29, Odense C DK-5000, Denmark.
E-mail address: pfhc@rsyd.dk

Wagner, Jr, by means of macroaggregated albumin,[3,4] the diagnosis of acute myocardial infarction in the 1970s by ^{99m}Tc stanneous pyrophosphate and ^{201}Tl,[5,6] radionuclide ventriculography for the measurement of ventricular function and not least myocardial perfusion scintigraphy with ^{201}Tl or with ^{99m}Tc-labeled compounds,[7–9] PET perfusion imaging using ^{15}O-water, the gold standard of perfusion measurement, as well as ^{82}Rb and ^{13}NH$_3$ and in recent years ^{18}F-labelled PET probes targeting mitochondrial complex 1.[10,11] At this point, molecular imaging has been in use for decades in the assessment of cardiac viability, sarcoidosis, and amyloidosis, as well as for the diagnosis of cardiovascular infection, inflammation, and neoplasm.[12]

Nonetheless, molecular imaging stands to lose ground in various clinical applications, including the study of myocardial perfusion in patients with angina pectoris and serial measurement of left ventricular ejection fraction during cancer chemotherapy. The task of ruling out significant coronary artery disease has successfully been taken over by cardiac computed tomography (CT) scans,[13,14] leaving perfusion studies for assessment of the clinical significance of CT-proven coronary artery disease.[15–17] Smart 3-dimensional echocardiographic measurements of left ventricular ejection fraction are much faster and cheaper, although less reliable, than multigated radioisotope determination. In addition, echocardiography provides significant information regarding the diastolic function and regional contraction pattern that is not that easily obtained with radionuclide techniques.[18,19]

However, molecular imaging in CVD offers entirely new options in the study and management of atherosclerosis, the most common cause of death in the United States[20] and, according to the World Health Organization, the world's number one killer.[21] Most initiatives intended to alleviate the human and economic costs of this disease are aimed at controlling risk factors and improving primary care of CVD management. Modern PET molecular imaging plays a complementary and innovative role by focusing on early disease, when the chance of cure or effective control may be significantly greater. The basis for this shift was laid 17 years ago with the first reported use of FDG for assessment of arterial wall inflammation,[22,23] followed almost a decade later by the introduction of NaF-PET for imaging of molecular arterial wall calcification.[24–31] More recent experience suggests that the potential value of PET imaging in atherosclerosis is not primarily a matter of diagnosing or characterizing the vulnerable plaque,[32,33] because the clinical significance of this approach may be less than anticipated. Rather, the main focus should be on measuring the atherosclerotic burden and its activity in the body,[34] preferably as early as possible in the course of the disease.

MOLECULAR IMAGING OF ATHEROSCLEROSIS

Traditionally, the atherosclerotic process has been considered a product of inflammation mobilizing monocytes, which differentiate into macrophages and become foam cells by phagocytizing lipids, particularly low-density lipoproteins.[35,36] Along with cellular debris, these foam cells form the main part of the atherosclerotic plaque. At the center of these plaques is a necrotic core that holds minute vesicles giving rise to microcalcification, which can contribute to plaque rupture (**Fig. 1**), but can also stabilize the plaque once inflammation subsides and overt macrocalcification takes

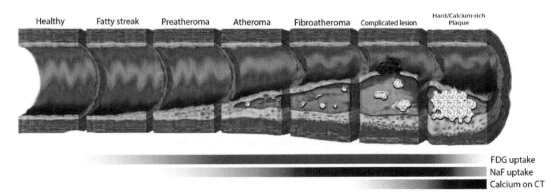

Fig. 1. Progression from healthy to hard calcium-rich arterial wall lesion. ^{18}F-fluorodeoxyglucose (FDG) and ^{18}F-sodium fluoride (NaF) uptakes precede vascular calcification evident on computed tomography scans. The stronger predictive power of NaF uptake and the identification of active calcification by NaF PET herald a paradigm shift in atherosclerosis imaging. (*Courtesy of* Reza Piri, MD, Odense, Denmark.)

over.[37,38] This complicated line of processes with multiple modifying and contributing factors has given rise to a number of gamma camera and PET tracers targeting features of the atherosclerotic plaque, including inflammatory cells, lipids and fatty acids, hypoxia, angiogenesis, proteases, thrombosis, apoptosis, and microcalcification, as recently summarized by Nakahara and colleagues.[36] To these might be added matrix metalloproteinases tagged with ^{111}In, ^{99m}Tc, ^{123}I, and [18]F[39] and more recently ^{18}F-fluorinated matrix metalloproteinase inhibitors[40] and [89]Zr-labeled high-density lipoprotein forming natural nanoparticles that have been shown to accumulate in advanced atherosclerotic lesions of established animal atherosclerosis models.[41] However, practically none of the potentially more specific radiopharmaceuticals have attained extensive human use. The notable exceptions are the rather unspecific, but much more common tracers FDG and NaF, whose full potential in this application is not yet known.

PET WITH ^{18}F-FLUORODEOXYGLUCOSE/ COMPUTED TOMOGRAPHY SCANS IN ATHEROSCLEROSIS
Vulnerable Plaque

Multiple efforts with multiple modalities including PET have been made to identify features of the vulnerable plaque with the purpose of predicting the risk of future cardiovascular events.[36] Clinical studies in patients with stable cancer have shown that increased FDG uptake in plaques in major arteries and the carotid arteries is associated with a higher risk of cardiovascular and cerebrovascular events, respectively.[42,43] However, as pointed out by Dilsizian and Jadvar,[44] FDG uptake may not be able to differentiate morphologically unstable (inflammatory) from stable (noninflammatory) atherosclerotic plaque, and there are other vascular diseases in which macrophages and inflammation play an important role in the absence of atherosclerosis (eg, Takayasu arteritis, chemotherapy- or radiation-induced vascular inflammation, and foreign body reactions such as synthetic arterial graft), meaning that "the nonspecific nature of FDG uptake by any cell (upregulated under hypoxic conditions or other microenvironmental factors)" calls for caution "when interpreting vascular FDG uptake as indicative of inflammatory atherosclerosis in the clinical setting."[44] These results and results obtained recently by our group challenge some of the preliminary conclusions that we drew in a prior review, including that, by targeting macrophages and hypoxia, FDG PET can "potentially detect

atherosclerosis, evaluate response to treatment, and prognosticate risk for acute cardiovascular events," and further that arterial FDG uptake is "helpful in risk stratification of patients at risk for CVD, beyond standard tools, such as the Framingham risk score (FRS) and coronary calcium score."[45] As argued in a review by Arbab-Zadeh and Fuster,[34] multiple pathologic and clinical studies suggest that the vulnerable plaque is more a myth than a reality of clinical significance and that the quest to identify vulnerable atherosclerotic plaques may be quixotic. Their more cogent arguments include (a) numerous investigations have demonstrated that many (if not most) plaques rupture without clinical symptoms, (b) the percentage of patients with subclinical plaque ruptures varies vastly depending on the risk profile and assessment methods, (c) plaque rupture and healing are frequently clinically silent, (d) millions of individuals most likely unknowingly experience plaque rupture each year, (e) plaque morphology changes in the span of months, gaining or losing their vulnerable characteristics, and (f) in patients with acute coronary syndrome, plaque rupture is frequently found in nonculprit lesions. The authors propose that a state of generalized vulnerability is more important than the individual sites of vulnerability in a patient. Very few plaque ruptures will trigger symptomatic events; therefore, the prediction of adverse outcome based on characteristics of particular lesions is "unlikely to be of incremental benefit for risk prediction over established risk factors (eg, extent and distribution of atherosclerotic plaque burden).[34]

We agree with this assertion from a molecular imaging perspective. PET scans can measure the extent and severity of atherosclerotic burden in an organ or the entire body and provide a global disease score, which we consider a conceptually more correct expression of the disease and its activity than sequential examinations of a few selected lesions.[28,46,47] With FDG PET, it is possible to demonstrate the presence of inflammation with a reproducibility that seems to be sufficient to allow demonstration of spontaneous or disease-inflicted changes. However, the question of whether this inflammation precedes or follows the formation of atherosclerotic calcification remains unanswered.[48]

Relation to Risk Factors

In their 2001 study of 137 patients undergoing either whole body or lower extremity FDG PET scans, Yun and colleagues[22] demonstrated that one-half of all participants had abnormal FDG uptake in at least one of the following studied arteries: abdominal aorta, iliac, proximal femoral, and popliteal arteries (34% of patients aged 20–40 years, 50% of patients aged 41–60 years, and 61% of patients aged 61–80 years). Since then, a number of studies of various designs applying different imaging techniques and vastly differing image analyses have demonstrated similar findings,[23–27,49–55] often showing "strong" or "highly significant" correlations between age and risk factors. Dependency on age is also what we see with extended analyses[55–58] of the CAMONA (Cardiovascular Molecular Calcification Assessed by ^{18}F-NaF PET/CT) study in Odense, Denmark, in which a total of 139 participants aged 21 to 75 years, 52% men (89 healthy controls and 50 patients with angina pectoris) were examined with both FDG and NaF PET/CT scans.[59] However, with modern imaging acquisition and analysis techniques, we and others could not demonstrate a significant correlation of thoracic aortic FDG uptake and the 10-year FRS, whereas this was clearly present between NaF uptake and the FRS (Fig. 2).[59,60] The many analyses we have performed on our CAMONA material, or part of it, have without gender differences shown frequent and higher FDG uptake in the thoracic aorta and its 3 segments in patients with angina pectoris than in healthy controls and weak but positive correlation with age, which is also more pronounced in patients versus controls.[55,56] We found the same tendencies in the abdominal aorta,[57] but not in the carotid arteries.[58]

It is difficult to compare the many reports on FDG uptake in the arterial system owing to vast differences in design and materials, frequent use of retrospective data and post hoc analyzes, and above all a lack of standardization with regard to image acquisition, analysis, and interpretation. In reviewing 49 articles, Huet and colleagues[61] found 53 different acquisition protocols, 51 reconstruction protocols, and 46 quantification methods to characterize atherosclerotic lesions on FDG PET scans.

Despite the variability in the methodology, the evidence suggests that foci of increased FDG uptake are frequently present in major arteries of the body and that this tendency increases slightly with age, albeit with large interindividual differences, and that there seems to be only a vague association between arterial FDG uptake and cardiovascular risk factors.

Monitoring of Treatment

Preclinical studies in hyperlipidemic rabbits have demonstrated a decrease in aortic FDG uptake and macrophage infiltration of the aorta after antioxidant therapy[62] and an increase in aortic FDG uptake in rabbits on a sustained atherogenic diet.[63] In the few human studies on the role of FDG PET in monitoring the effects of statins, Tahara and colleagues[64] demonstrated a decrease in FDG uptakes in the thoracic aorta and/or carotid arteries after 3 months of therapy, whereas Ishii and colleagues[65] reported a decrease in FDG target-to-background ratio (TBR) in the ascending aorta and femoral arteries after atorvastatin 20 mg for 6 months. Finally, in a randomized trial including 76 patients with known atherosclerosis, Tawakol and colleagues[66] found reductions in arterial FDG activity after 4 and 12 weeks of treatment with both 10 and 80 mg of

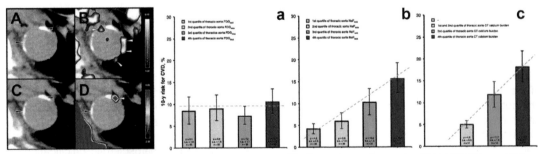

Fig. 2. (Left) Axial computed tomography (CT) scan (A, C), ^{18}F-fluorodeoxyglucose (FDG) PET/CT (B), and ^{18}F-sodium fluoride (NaF) PET/CT (D) images obtained at the same location in 69-year-old man with hypertension, a body mass index of 28 kg/m[2], and a Framingham risk score of 26%. FDG accumulation is seen in the descending thoracic aorta (B, white arrowheads), but not at sites with structural calcium deposits (A, C, black arrowheads). In the NaF PET/CT image (D), active (white arrowhead) and indolent (black arrowhead) vascular calcifications are distinguished. (Right) The estimated 10-year Framingham risk score in relation to quartiles of (a) thoracic aorta FDG activity, (b) thoracic aorta NaF activity, and (c) thoracic aorta CT calcium burden. Cardiovascular disease (CVD) risk is similar in all quartiles of thoracic aorta FDG activity, but increases linearly with each increasing quartile of thoracic aorta NaF uptake (P<.001 for a linear trend) and with each increasing quartile of thoracic aorta CT calcium burden (P<.001 for a linear trend). s.e., standard error; μ, mean.

atorvastatin, and a further decrease in the 80 mg group only after 12 weeks. Other antiatherosclerotic drugs have been evaluated by FDG PET imaging, however, without showing significant effects.[45]

Disease Progression

Of great scientific interest and potential clinical significance is the existence of a causal and/or temporal association between arterial wall inflammation and calcification. It remains unclear which of these processes precedes the other, to what extent they overlap or succeed each other in time and location, and whether or not they stimulate or inhibit each other and/or other elements of the atherosclerotic process. Relatively few studies have reported findings from 2 or more succeeding scans and none of them were designed to study disease progression.

Meirelles and colleagues[52] reviewed retrospectively the records of 100 consecutive patients with cancer (51 male, 49 female; aged 20–80 years) with at least 2 FDG PET/CT scans performed a mean of 7 months apart (range, 21 days to 3 years) and found aortic uptake in 70%, which had changed on the second scan in 55% of patients. Calcifications were often seen in patients with FDG uptake, but were present at the same site in only 2 cases, a finding that has been documented in several prior studies.[49,67,68] Calcification and FDG uptake correlated with age, and patients with diabetes, hypertension, hyperlipidemia, or a history of CVD had significantly more calcification. Calcifications were stable, but the fact that FDG uptake changed in more than one-half of patients led the authors to conclude that "inflammation in atheroma is a waxing and waning inflammatory process."[52]

Abdelbaky and colleagues[69] retrospectively studied 137 patients (aged 61 ± 13 years, 48.1% men) with inactive cancer, who underwent 2 or more FDG PET/CT examinations spaced 1 to 5 years apart. Using "square root-transformed difference of calcium volume score, with a cutoff value of 2.5" to determine whether vascular segments showed evidence of calcification, 67 aortic segments (9%) were deemed to have developed calcification. Baseline FDG uptake proved predictive of which patient would go on to develop calcification. In univariate analysis, segment standardized uptake value (SUV), segment TBR, age, hyperlipidemia, statin therapy, systolic blood pressure, baseline CVD, and follow-up duration were all associated with subsequent calcium deposition, which led to the conclusion that "arterial inflammation precedes subsequent [calcium] deposition, a marker of plaque progression, within

the underlying location in the artery wall."[69] Hetterich and colleagues[70] retrospectively studied scans of 94 patients, aged 62.5 ± 8.7 years, 35% men, who underwent FDG PET/CT scans at baseline and at follow-up 14.5 ± 3.5 months later because of various known or suspected cancers. Annualized calcified plaque volume, judged by the Agatston score, increased by 10% in the carotid arteries, by 23%, 16%, and 18% in the thoracic, abdominal, and entire aorta, respectively, and by 9% in the iliac arteries. The lumen area measured in the carotids and the aorta decreased by 10% and 2%, respectively. Interestingly, FDG uptake, quantified by the TBR, did not change at all in any of these locations, and hypertension and not FGD uptake was the only independent predictor of calcification. In a post hoc analysis of 130 patients in the del-PLAQUE trial, Joshi and colleagues[71] found no effect of dalcetrapib on vessel wall inflammation. This analysis revealed that patients with a zero calcium score at baseline had almost no new calcification at follow-up, whereas patients with a nonzero baseline calcium score had a higher rate of calcification, a tendency that was most pronounced in the aortic arch. However, no relationship was noted between baseline calcification and change in inflammation.[71] Cho and colleagues[72] analyzed data from 96 asymptomatic middle-aged participants (84% men) without a history of cardiac disease, who underwent FDG PET/CT scans and CT calcium scoring on the same day and had follow-up scans 1 or more years later (mean, 4.3 years) without having suffered interim cardiac events or received statin therapy in between. Their aim was to investigate whether FDG uptake in the carotid arteries, ascending aorta, and abdominal aorta can predict coronary artery calcification progression in asymptomatic individuals. At baseline, 21 participants (22%) had coronary artery calcification by CT scanning, whereas 75 participants (78%) did not, and 59 of these participants (79%) had no coronary artery calcification at follow-up. Coronary artery calcification progression was observed in 31 participants (32%), in 15 of 21 participants (76%) with coronary artery calcification at baseline, and in 16 of 75 participants (21%) without coronary artery calcification at baseline. FDG uptake was significantly higher in coronary artery calcification progressors, and significant positive correlations were observed between several FDG uptake parameters and coronary artery calcification progression, but all of them far too weak to allow relevant prediction. Interestingly, in multivariate analysis, only peak TBR for FDG uptake in the abdominal aorta was significantly associated with coronary artery calcification progression.[72]

None of these studies showed a close association in time and place between arterial wall FDG uptake and arterial wall (macro)calcification, only a vague relationship that is moderately more pronounced with age but lacks striking coincidence or covariation. A picture emerges of macrocalcification visible on CT scans, which changes little over time, whereas FDG uptake changes rapidly ("waxing and waning") with regard to location, size, and intensity. On the whole, these sequential studies are difficult to interpret, because they were not planned as prospective trials with a primary focus on changes in FDG uptake and calcification and because they lack sufficient follow-up.

In conclusion, FDG uptake in the arterial system is a frequent finding that, unlike CT-visible macrocalcification, varies rapidly over time. It is positively, but vaguely, associated with age, it overlaps with arterial wall macrocalcifications only to a limited degree, and it cannot with any reasonable certainty predict progression of arterial macrocalcifications. It remains unknown if it is always a predecessor of arterial wall microcalcification and/or macrocalcification.

18F-SODIUM FLUORIDE PET/COMPUTED TOMOGRAPHY SCANS IN ATHEROSCLEROSIS
Vulnerable Plaque

Molecular mechanisms of NaF deposition in bone have been summarized by Czernin and colleagues[73] In short, NaF is taken up by bone after a single pass of blood, so that the initial NaF distribution reflects blood flow that varies among different bones. Otherwise, NaF is rapidly cleared from plasma and excreted by the kidneys, leaving less than 10% in plasma after 1 hour and less than 3% after 5 hours. After chemisorption onto hydroxyapatite, ^{18}F exchanges rapidly for OH on the surface of a hydroxyapatite matrix to form fluoroapatite, the first part of this process being rapid (seconds, minutes), the last part slow (days, weeks).[74–76] If the uptake of NaF by the arterial wall can be explained by a similar mechanism, NaF would presumably be taken up rapidly by microcalcification in the necrotic core of focal arterial injuries irrespective of whether this process is preceded by focal inflammation. NaF PET does not suffer from the same disadvantage as FDG PET in atherosclerosis imaging, namely, that physiologic myocardial glucose metabolism precludes imaging of coronary artery inflammation. In contrast, quantification of arterial wall uptake of NaF PET is challenged by spillover from nearby bones, which makes it difficult to determine blood background activity.[77]

Few studies have examined the potential significance of NaF uptake for characterizing vulnerable plaques. Joshi and colleagues[32] found that 93% of patients after a myocardial infarction had higher NaF uptake in culprit versus nonculprit coronary lesions, that marked NaF uptake was present at the site of all carotid plaque ruptures, and that nearly one-half of patients with stable angina had plaques with focal NaF uptake that were associated with more high-risk features on intravascular ultrasound examination than those without NaF uptake. Irkle and colleagues[78] used electron microscopy, autoradiography, histology, and PET/CT scans to show that NaF adsorbs to calcified deposits within plaque with high affinity and is selective and specific in a way that NaF PET/CT imaging can distinguish between areas of macrocalcification and microcalcification. Finally, Marchesseau and colleagues[79] reported increased NaF uptake in coronary culprit lesions in a small cohort of patients after a myocardial infarction and noted that NaF was taken up by scarred myocardial tissue, a finding that is reminiscent of the earlier work of Bonte and colleagues,[5] who visualized acute myocardial infarction using ^{99m}Tc-pyrophosphate scintigraphy. However, the characterization of vulnerable plaques may prove less clinically useful than imagined; as argued by Arbab-Zadeh and Fuster,[34] the question remains of what should be the preferred measure of atherosclerosis: the atherosclerotic burden, its location, extent and activity, or something else?

Relation to Risk Factors and Treatment

As described, arterial wall uptake of NaF correlates not only with age, but contrary to FDG, consistently also with risk factors for atherosclerosis and CVD.[25,29,55–59] From the information collected thus far, it seems that NaF PET reflects key elements of initiation and development of the atherosclerotic process in a way that makes it worthwhile to explore its potential for studying the effects of antiatherosclerotic treatment.

Disease Progression

NaF-PET may be a better indicator of atherosclerotic disease progression than FDG PET. Studies of the latter have been heterogeneous and often difficult to interpret, but have generally portrayed arterial FDG uptake as "waxing and waning" and only rarely overlapping with NaF uptake. This observation raises questions about the ability of FDG to predict or indicate more than local waxing and waning arterial inflammation, especially because it seems that there is no direct link between focal inflammation and microcalcification.

It seems more likely that such a link exists between microcalcification and macrocalcification. This relationship has not been reported yet. What we have seen so far from data of the CAMONA study is a more tight relationship between NaF uptake and risk factors than between FDF uptake and risk factors,[55–58,80–86] a finding that supports the assumption that NaF uptake may be a more faithful real-time representative of early active calcification. However, only carefully conducted longitudinal studies will reveal if this notion is correct.

Animal Studies

Studies applying an Ossabaw miniature swine model of the metabolic syndrome have demonstrated that NaF uptake in the coronary arteries precedes the emergence of macroscopic calcification on intravascular ultrasound and CT scans.[87–89] When fed a high-calorie atherogenic diet and forced to live a sedentary lifestyle, the Ossabaw swine develops progressive coronary artery disease from the stages of clinically insignificant fatty streaks through necrotic, flow-limiting lesions with macrocalcification detectable by intravascular ultrasound examination.[90] Comparing lean pigs and pigs with the metabolic syndrome without evidence of coronary artery calcification by CT scans, quantitative PET imaging showed almost a 2.5 higher NaF uptake in the hearts of pigs with the metabolic syndrome compared with lean pigs.[89] Another preclinical PET/CT study demonstrated that increased ^{18}F-NaF uptake in coronary arteries is a biomarker for early coronary artery calcification in pigs with coronary artery disease that lack frank evidence of calcification by intravascular ultrasound and CT imaging.[91] These findings imply that ^{18}F-NaF binds to microcalcifications too small to be detected using anatomic or morphologic imaging modalities, an interpretation that is strengthened by histopathology data revealing sparse calcifications within the proximal region of the coronary artery. These data do not significantly correlate with ^{18}F-NaF uptake in the coronary arteries, suggesting that histologic assessment detects macroaggregates of hydroxyapatite, but not the microcalcifications visualized by ^{18}F-NaF PET/CT scans.[92] Several findings in this type of preclinical swine model of coronary artery disease have hinted at a role for ^{18}F-NaF PET/CT scans in the early detection of atherosclerosis.[58,59] With regard to treatment, Lee et al[93] have demonstrated almost complete attenuation by atorvastatin of coronary disease in diabetic dyslipidemic swine, a finding that has thus far not been verified in humans.

PET/MRI IN ATHEROSCLEROSIS

Hybrid PET/MRI has been applied in experimental animal studies of atherosclerotic plaques that have used FDG and other tracers, including nanoparticles.[94–96] PET/MRI studies of atherosclerosis in humans remain sparse and are largely limited to first-in-human or feasibility studies.[97–100] Of particular interest is an observational, longitudinal, and prospective cohort study by Fernández-Ortiz and colleagues[101] comprising a target population of 4000 healthy participants (40–54 years old, 35% women) based in Madrid, Spain. In a subgroup of 1300 participants with evidence of atherosclerosis on 2-dimensional/3-dimensional ultrasound examination or cardiac CT scans, FDG PET/MRI of the carotid and iliofemoral arteries was performed at baseline and repeated at 3 and 6 years. At the 3-year mark, the authors found that subclinical atherosclerosis—classified as focal (1 site affected), intermediate (2–3 sites), or generalized (4–6 sites)—was present in 63% of participants (71% of men, 48% of women) and that 41% had intermediate and generalized atherosclerosis. Plaques were most common in the iliofemorals (44%), carotids (31%), and aorta (25%). Coronary artery calcification was present in only 18% of cases. Among participants with a low 10-year FRS, subclinical disease was present in 58%.[102] It will be highly interesting to learn the result of the baseline FDG PET/MRI scans and to what degree these may have changed after 6 years.

LIMITATIONS AND CAVEATS

Despite the unique advantages of PET, many of which have been mentioned herein, it is appropriate to summarize the main caveats and limitations, which need to be considered to get the best out of this technology. The spatial resolution of PET is limited to a few millimeters under optimized conditions, but is actually closer to 5 to 10 mm in practice. This is due to blurring of imaging from patient, cardiac, and respiratory motion, some of which is irregular and nonepisodic in nature and cannot be accurately corrected for by current techniques. Therefore, the higher sensitivity of PET may not be fully used without being paired with the much better spatial solution of CT scans and MRI. The latter 2 methods can determine with very high precision the location of an abnormal weak signal that only PET can capture. CT scans and MRI suffer from insufficient sensitivity, which means that they may ignore weak signals, even if abnormal. Moreover, they detect mostly anatomic, morphologic, or structural changes in tissues and organs that typically occur late in the disease process. This principle applies to metastatic cancer[103] and most likely to atherosclerosis as well. Other considerations include motion artifacts and partial volume effects, and have been the focus of prior studies.[46,47,104] Finally, the choice of parameter—TBR, SUV, metabolic tumor volume, or another local or global metric[28,47,80,83,92]—can greatly affect the interpretation of a PET study. Ideally, PET parameters should be standardized and automated for ease of clinical use.

CONSIDERATIONS ABOUT ATHEROSCLEROTIC DISEASE

Most of what we know about atherosclerosis is based on histologic examination and experimental animal models of atherosclerosis rather than in vivo human studies. The results of FDG and NaF PET imaging of atherosclerosis are often in conflict and make it difficult to spot the more important underlying mechanisms and establish a unifying concept that can provide the basis for research into and improved management of this condition. From FDG PET imaging, it seems that focal arterial wall inflammation arises in response to minor injuries, most of which are harmless and

heal quickly without any long-term damage. However, a subset of injuries, whether by virtue of their location, severity, or other characteristics, cause lasting damage to the arterial wall. Whether this process begins with an inflammatory cascade that culminates in apoptosis, necrosis, and calcification, or rather that calcifications arise at areas of stress (eg, aortic arch or bifurcation) and induce chronic calcification and plaque formation, is not yet clear. To best apply PET imaging in atherosclerosis, it will be important to determine whether arterial wall microcalcification by NaF PET imaging is (i) always a forerunner to CT-visible macrocalcification, (ii) always an indicator of active, ongoing arterial wall calcification, (iii) comparable or superior to other known risk factors, and (iv) able to reliably monitor response to antiatherosclerotic therapy. If NaF PET imaging possesses most of these key features, it may replace other modalities in current use for patients with CVD even though it is more costly and less accessible.

WHERE TO GO FROM HERE

NaF PET imaging may cause a shift from the management of the late occurring symptomatic effects

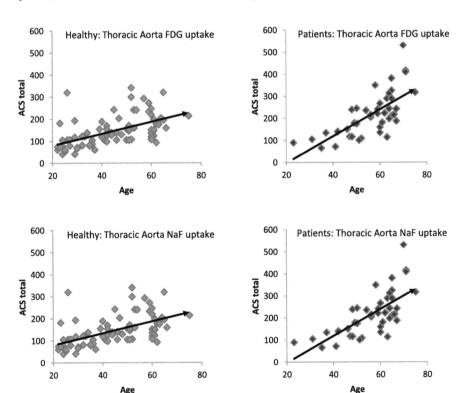

Fig. 3. Significant correlation of 18F-sodium fluoride (NaF) uptake and age in the thoracic aorta of healthy subjects (*left*) and angina pectoris patients (*right*). Note the large scatter meaning that, for instance, a young and healthy control participant may have as high or higher uptake than an old patient and vice versa.

of atherosclerosis to the early detection and quantification of arterial wall microcalcification in asymptomatic participants long before macrocalcification has developed and become detectable on CT scans. Traditionally, it may have been viewed as unorthodox to search for disease before the onset of symptoms and functional impairment. However, with modern technology, this outdated viewpoint need no longer apply. In cardiology, we have been testing for hypercholesterolemia and hypertension in asymptomatic patients on a massive scale for decades, ever since inexpensive testing became easily accessible. The downside has been enormous drug expenditures and side effects as a result of millions of people being put on lifelong treatment on the basis of a few cheap measurements and statistical evidence that did not necessarily apply to each individual patient. Molecular imaging, including NaF PET/CT scanning, offers more individualized disease assessment than what we are used to, particularly in the early stages of disease. From analyses of the CAMONA data, we know now that there is a positive correlation between age and the uptake of NaF in the heart (ie, coronary arteries), thoracic and abdominal aorta, carotids, and choroid plexus in the brain. We also note that the slope of the regression line in all locations is modest, although greater in patients than controls.[80–86] Furthermore, the individual differences are huge, meaning that some healthy volunteers and some patients with angina pectoris above the age of 70 may still have a very low atherosclerotic burden, whereas some symptomless young individuals already have significant arterial wall microcalcification (**Fig. 3**). In these parts of the arterial system, the Alavi-Carlsen global molecular calcium score, which is a measure of the total NaF uptake in part of the arterial system,[83,85] was a stronger predictor of the 10-year FRS than the commonly used parameters of average maximum SUV and average mean SUV. FDG uptake in these segments was positively correlated with age in patients only, but not with the 10-year FRS.[80–86] All positive correlations had a wide scatter (see **Fig. 3**), illustrating the need to characterize each individual participant by NaF PET imaging. Similarly, the scatter around the regression line when looking at the association with age was also so large that it questions the often postulated close association of atherosclerosis with age.

SUMMARY

What has been published thus far in the literature on the use of PET in atherosclerosis portends great clinical utility but leaves ambiguous as to how the modality will be applied. A case can be made for NaF PET emerging as the key technique for the early detection and grading of atherosclerosis when it is still symptomless and devoid of CT-detectable macrocalcification. Intervening at this early stage should produce a more efficacious response to therapy than later in the disease course when symptoms have appeared and organ damage has occurred. If this holds true, NaF PET imaging can be expected to play an increasingly central role in the diagnosis and management of atherosclerotic disease in the years to come.

REFERENCES

1. Blumgart HL, Yens OC. Studies on the velocity of blood flow: I. The method utilized. J Clin Invest 1926;4:1–13.
2. Patton DD. The birth of nuclear medicine instrumentation: Blumgart and Yens, 1925. J Nucl Med 2003;44:1362–5.
3. Potchen EJ. Reflections on the early years in nuclear medicine. Radiology 2000;214:623–9.
4. Wagner HN Jr, Sabiston DC Jr, McAfee JG, et al. Diagnosis of massive pulmonary embolism in man by radioisotope scanning. N Engl J Med 1964;271:377–83.
5. Bonte FJ, Parkey RW, Graham KD, et al. A new method for radionuclide imaging of myocardial infarcts. Radiology 1974;110:473–4.
6. Wackers FJ, Schoot JB, Sokole EB, et al. Noninvasive visualization of acute myocardial infarction in man with thallium-201. Br Heart J 1975;37:741–4.
7. Pitt B, Strauss HW. Myocardial imaging in the noninvasive evaluation of patients with suspected ischemic heart disease. Am J Cardiol 1976;37:797–806.
8. Strauss HW, Pitt B. Common procedures for the noninvasive determination of regional myocardial perfusion, evaluation of regional wall motion and detection of acute infarction. Am J Cardiol 1976;38:731–8.
9. Pitt B, Strauss HW. Myocardial perfusion imaging and gated cardiac blood pool scanning: clinical application. Am J Cardiol 1976;38:739–46.
10. Bergmann SR, Herrero P, Markham J, et al. Noninvasive quantitation of myocardial blood flow in human subjects with oxygen-15-labeled water and positron emission tomography. J Am Coll Cardiol 1989;14:639–52.
11. Maddahi J, Packard RRS. Cardiac PET perfusion tracers: current status and future directions. Semin Nucl Med 2014;44:333–43.
12. Dibble EH, Yoo DC. Precision medicine and PET/computed tomography in cardiovascular disorders. PET Clin 2017;12:459–73.

13. Takx RA, Blomberg BA, El Aidi H, et al. Diagnostic accuracy of stress myocardial perfusion imaging compared to invasive coronary angiography with fractional flow reserve meta-analysis. Circ Cardiovasc Imaging 2015;8(1) [pii:e002666].

14. Sørgaard MH, Kofoed KF, Linde JJ, et al. Diagnostic accuracy of static CT perfusion for the detection of myocardial ischemia. A systematic review and meta-analysis. J Cardiovasc Comput Tomogr 2016;10:450–7.

15. Thomassen A, Petersen H, Diederichsen ACP, et al. Hybrid CT angiography and quantitative 15O-water PET for assessment of coronary artery disease: comparison with quantitative coronary angiography. Eur J Nucl Med Mol Imaging 2013;40:1894–904.

16. Danad I, Raijmakers PG, Driessen RS, et al. Comparison of coronary CT angiography, SPECT, PET, and hybrid imaging for diagnosis of ischemic heart disease determined by fractional Flow reserve. JAMA Cardiol 2017;2:1100–7.

17. Thomassen A, Braad PE, Pedersen KT, et al. 15-O-water myocardial flow reserve PET and CT angiography by full hybrid PET/CT as a potential alternative to invasive angiography. Int J Cardiovasc Imaging 2018. https://doi.org/10.1007/s10554-018-1420-3.

18. Cameli M, Mondillo S, Solari M, et al. Echocardiographic assessment of left ventricular systolic function: from ejection fraction to torsion. Heart Fail Rev 2016;21:77–94.

19. Spitzer E, Ren B, Zijlstra F, et al. The role of automated 3D echocardiography for left ventricular ejection fraction assessment. Card Fail Rev 2017;3:97–101.

20. Heidenreich PA, Trogdon JG, Khavjou OA, et al. Forecasting the future of cardiovascular disease in the United States: a policy statement from the American Heart Association. Circulation 2011;123:933–44.

21. Worlds Health Organization. Cardiovascular disease. Available at: http://www.who.int/cardiovascular_diseases/en/. Accessed July 26, 2018.

22. Yun M, Yeh D, Araujo LI, et al. F-18 FDG uptake in the large arteries: a new observation. Clin Nucl Med 2001;26:314–9.

23. Yun M, Jang S, Cucchiara A, et al. 18F FDG uptake in the large arteries: a correlation study with the atherogenic risk factors. Semin Nucl Med 2002;32:70–6.

24. Derlin T, Richter U, Bannas P, et al. Feasibility of 18F-sodium fluoride PET/CT for imaging of atherosclerotic plaque. J Nucl Med 2010;51:862–5.

25. Derlin T, Wisotzki C, Richter U, et al. In vivo imaging of mineral deposition in carotid plaque using 18F-sodium fluoride PET/CT: correlation with atherogenic risk factors. J Nucl Med 2011;52:362–8.

26. Beheshti M, Saboury B, Mehta NN, et al. Detection and global quantification of cardiovascular molecular calcification by fluoro18-fluoride positron emission tomography/computed tomography–a novel concept. Hell J Nucl Med 2011;14:114–20.

27. Li Y, Berenji GR, Shaba WF, et al. Association of vascular fluoride uptake with vascular calcification and coronary artery disease. Nucl Med Commun 2012;33:14–20.

28. Basu S, Høilund-Carlsen PF, Alavi A. Assessing global cardiovascular molecular calcification with 18 F-fluoride PET/CT: will this become a clinical reality and a challenge to CT calcification scoring? Eur J Nucl Med Mol Imaging 2012;39:660–4.

29. Janssen T, Bannas P, Herrmann J, et al. Association of linear 18F-sodium fluoride accumulation in femoral arteries as a measure of diffuse calcification with cardiovascular risk factors: a PET/CT study. J Nucl Cardiol 2013;20:569–77.

30. Blomberg BA, Thomassen A, Takx RA, et al. Delayed sodium 18F-fluoride PET/CT imaging does not improve quantification of vascular calcification metabolism: results from the CAMONA study. J Nucl Cardiol 2014;21:293–304.

31. Blomberg BA, Thomassen A, Takx RA, et al. Delayed 18F-fluorodeoxyglucose PET/CT imaging Improves quantification of atherosclerotic plaque inflammation: results from the CAMONA Study. J Nucl Cardiol 2014;21:588–97.

32. Joshi NV, Vesey AT, Williams MC, et al. 18 F-fluoride positron emission tomography for identification of ruptured and high-risk coronary atherosclerotic plaques: a prospective clinical trial. Lancet 2014;383:705–13.

33. Lee JM, Bang JI, Koo BK, et al. Clinical relevance of 18F-sodium fluoride positron-emission tomography in noninvasive identification of high-risk plaque in patients with coronary artery disease. Circ Cardiovasc Imaging 2017;10(11) [pii:e006704].

34. Arbab-Zadeh A, Fuster V. The myth of the "vulnerable plaque": transitioning from a focus on individual lesions to atherosclerotic disease burden for coronary artery disease risk assessment. J Am Coll Cardiol 2015;65:846–55.

35. Nakahara T, Strauss HW. From inflammation to calcification in atherosclerosis. Eur J Nucl Med Mol Imaging 2017;44:858–60.

36. Nakahara T, Narula J, Strauss HW. Molecular imaging of vulnerable plaque. Semin Nucl Med 2018;48:291–8.

37. Lee SE, Chang HJ, Sung JM, et al. Effects of statins on coronary atherosclerotic plaques: the PRADIGM (progression of atherosclerotic plague determined by computed tomographic angiography imaging) study. JACC Cardiovasc Imaging 2018. https://doi.org/10.1016/j.jcmg.2018.04.015.

38. Andelius L, Mortensen MB, Nørgaard BL, et al. Impact of statin therapy on coronary plaque burden and composition assessed by coronary computed tomographic angiography: a systematic review and meta-analysis. Eur Heart J Cardiovasc Imaging 2018;19:850–8.

39. Matusiak N, van Waarde A, Bischoff R, et al. Probes for non-invasive matrix metalloproteinase-targeted imaging with PET and SPECT. Curr Pharm Des 2013;19:4647–72.

40. Butsch V, Börgel F, Galla F, et al. Design, (radio) synthesis, and in vitro and in vivo evaluation of highly selective and potent matrix metalloproteinase 12 (MMP-12) inhibitors as radiotracers for positron emission tomography. J Med Chem 2018;61:4115–34.

41. Pérez-Medina C, Binderup T, Lobatto ME, et al. In vivo PET imaging of high-density lipoprotein in multiple atherosclerosis models. JACC Cardiovasc Imaging 2016;9:950–61.

42. Marnane M, Merwick A, Sheehan OC, et al. Carotid plaque inflammation on 18F-fluorodeoxyglucose positron emission tomography predicts early stroke recurrence. Ann Neurol 2012;71:709–18.

43. Figueroa AL, Subramanian SS, Cury RC, et al. Distribution of inflammation within carotid atherosclerotic plaques with high-risk morphological features: a comparison between positron emission tomography activity, plaque morphology, and histopathology. Circ Cardiovasc Imaging 2012;5:69–77.

44. Dilsizian V, Jadvar H. Science to practice: does FDG differentiate morphologically unstable from stable atherosclerotic plaque? Radiology 2017;283:1–3.

45. Blomberg B, Høilund-Carlsen PF. [18F]-fluordeoxyglucose PET imaging of atherosclerosis. PET Clin 2015;10(1):1–7.

46. Alavi A, Werner TJ, Høilund-Carlsen PF. What can be and what cannot be accomplished with PET to detect and characterize atherosclerotic plaques. J Nucl Cardiol 2017. https://doi.org/10.1007/s12350-017-0977-x.

47. Alavi A, Werner TJ, Høilund-Carlsen PF. PET-based imaging to detect and characterize cardiovascular disorders: unavoidable path for the foreseeable future. J Nucl Cardiol 2018;25(1):203–7.

48. Nakahara T, Narula J, Strauss HW. Calcification and inflammation in atherosclerosis: which is the chicken, and which is the egg? J Am Coll Cardiol 2016;67(1):79–80.

49. Ben-Haim S, Kupzov E, Tamir A, et al. Evaluation of 18F-FDG uptake and arterial wall calcifications using 18F-FDG PET/CT. J Nucl Med 2004;45:1816–21.

50. Bural GG, Torigian DA, Chamroonrat W, et al. FDG-PET is an effective imaging modality to detect and

51. Rominger A, Saam T, Wolpers S, et al. 18F-FDG PET/CT identifies patients at risk for future vascular events in an otherwise asymptomatic cohort with neoplastic disease. J Nucl Med 2009;50:1611–20.

52. Meirelles GS, Gonen M, Strauss HW. 18F-FDG uptake and calcifications in thoracic aorta on positron emission tomography/computed tomography examinations: frequency and stability of serial scans. J Thorac Imaging 2011;26:54–62.

53. Strobl FF, Rominger A, Wolpers S, et al. Impact of cardiovascular risk factors on vessel wall inflammation and calcified plaque burden differs across vascular beds: a PET-CT study. Int J Cardiovasc Imaging 2013;29:1899–908.

54. Pasha AK, Moghbel M, Saboury B, et al. Effects of age and cardiovascular risk factors on (18) F-FDG PET/CT quantification of atherosclerosis in the aorta and peripheral arteries. Hell J Nucl Med 2014;18:5–10.

55. Blomberg BA, Thomassen A, de Jong PA, et al. Reference values for fluorine-18-fluorodeoxyglucose and fluorine-18-sodium fluoride uptake in human arteries: a prospective evaluation of 89 healthy adults. Nucl Med Commun 2017;38:998–1006.

56. Emamzadehfard S, Raynor W, Paydary K, et al. Evaluation of the role of age and cardiovascular risk factors on FDG-PET/CT quantification of atherosclerosis in the thoracic aorta [abstract]. J Nucl Med 2017;58(Suppl 1):1181.

57. Arani L, Gharavi M, Saboury B, et al. Assessment of the role of age and cardiovascular risk factors on 18F-Fluorodeoxyglucose (18F-FDG) and 18F-Sodium Fluoride (NaF) uptake in abdominal aortic artery [abstract]. J Nucl Med 2018;58(Suppl 1):1539.

58. Emamzadehfard S, Castro S, Werner T, et al. Does FDG PET/CT precisely detect carotid artery inflammation? [abstract]. J Nucl Med 2017;58(Suppl 1):1550.

59. Blomberg BA, de Jong PA, Thomassen A, et al. Thoracic aorta calcification but not inflammation is associated with increased cardiovascular disease risk: results of the CAMONA study. Eur J Nucl Med Mol Imaging 2017;44:249–58.

60. Morbelli S, Fiz F, Piccardo A, et al. Divergent determinants of 18F–NaF uptake and visible calcium deposition in large arteries: relationship with Framingham risk score. Int J Cardiovasc Imaging 2014;30:439–47.

61. Huet P, Burg S, Le Guludec D, et al. Variability and uncertainty of 18F-FDG PET imaging protocols for assessing inflammation in atherosclerosis: suggestions for improvements. J Nucl Med 2015;56:552–9.

62. Ogawa M, Magata Y, Kato T, et al. Application of 18F-FDG PET for monitoring the therapeutic effect non antiinflammatory drugs on stabilization of vulnerable atherosclerotic plaques. J Nucl Med 2006;47:1845–50.

63. Worthley SG, Zhang ZY, Machac J, et al. In vivo non-invasive serial monitoring of FDG-PET progression and regression in a rabbit model of atherosclerosis. Int J Cardiovasc Imaging 2009; 25:251–7.

64. Tahara N, Kai H, Ishibashi M, et al. Simvastatin attenuates plaque inflammation: evaluation by fluorodeoxyglucose positron emission tomography. J Am Coll Cardiol 2006;48:1825–31.

65. Ishii H, Nishio M, Takahashi H, et al. Comparison of atorvastatin 5 and 20 mg/d for reducing F-18 fluorodeoxyglucose uptake in atherosclerotic plaques on positron emission tomography/computed tomography: a randomized, investigator-blinded, open-label, 6-month study in Japanese adults scheduled for percutaneous coronary intervention. Clin Ther 2010;32:2337–47.

66. Tawakol A, Singh P, Rudd JH, et al. Effect of treatment for 12 weeks with rilapladib, a lipoprotein-associated phospholipase A2 inhibitor, on arterial inflammation as assessed with 18F-fluorodeoxyglucose-positron emission tomography imaging. J Am Coll Cardiol 2014;63:86–8.

67. Tatsumi M, Cohade C, Nakamoto Y, et al. Fluorodeoxyglucose uptake in the aortic wall at PET/CT: possible finding for active atherosclerosis 1. Radiology 2003;229:831–7.

68. Dunphy MP, Freiman A, Larson SM, et al. Association of vascular 18F-FDG uptake with vascular calcification. J Nucl Med 2005;46:1278–84.

69. Abdelbaky A, Corsini E, Figueroa AL, et al. Focal arterial inflammation precedes subsequent calcification in the same location: a longitudinal FDG-PET/CT study. Circ Cardiovasc Imaging 2013;6: 747–54.

70. Hetterich H, Rominger A, Walter L, et al. Natural history of atherosclerotic disease progression as assessed by (18)F-FDG PET/CT. Int J Cardiovasc Imaging 2016;32:49–59.

71. Joshi FR, Rajani NK, Abt M, et al. Does vascular calcification accelerate inflammation? A substudy of the dal-PLAQUE trial. J Am Coll Cardiol 2016; 67:69–78.

72. Cho SG, Park SK, Kim J, et al. Prediction of coronary calcium progression by FDG uptake of large arteries in asymptomatic individuals. Eur J Nucl Med Mol Imaging 2017;44:129–40.

73. Czernin J, Satyamurthy N, Schiepers C. Molecular mechanisms of bone 18F-NaF deposition. J Nucl Med 2010;51:1826–9.

74. Blau M, Ramanik G, Bender MA. ^{18}F-fluoride for bone imaging. Semin Nucl Med 1972;2:31–7.

75. Wootton R, Doré C. The single-passage extraction of 18F in rabbit bone. Clin Phys Physiol Meas 1986; 7:333–43.

76. Hawkins RA, Choi Y, Huang SC, et al. Evaluation of the skeletal kinetics of fluorine-18-fluoride ion with PET. J Nucl Med 1992;33:633–42.

77. Blomberg BA, Thomassen A, de Jong PA, et al. Impact of personal characteristics and technical factors on quantification of [18F]-sodium fluoride uptake in human arteries: prospective evaluation of healthy subjects. J Nucl Med 2015;56:1534–40.

78. Irkle A, Vesey AT, Lewis DY, et al. Identifying active vascular microcalcification by (18)F-sodium fluoride positron emission tomography. Nat Commun 2015;6:7495.

79. Marchesseau S, Seneviratna A, Sjoholm T, et al. Hybrid PET/CT and PET/MRI imaging of vulnerable coronary plaque and myocardial scar tissue in acute myocardial infarction. J Nucl Cardiol 2017. https://doi.org/10.1007/s12350-017-0918-8.

80. Paydary K, Emamzadehfard S, Gholami S, et al. 18F-NaF PET/CT quantification of vascular calcification in the thoracic aorta is associated with increasing age and presence of cardiovascular risk factors [abstract]. J Nucl Med 2017;58(Suppl 1):298.

81. Castro S, Acosta-Montenegro O, Muser D, et al. Association between common carotid artery molecular calcification assessed by 18F-NaF PET/CT and biomarkers of vulnerable atheromatous plaques: results from the CAMONA study [abstract]. J Nucl Med 2017;58(Suppl 1):443.

82. Castro S, Emamzadehfard S, Muser D, et al. Aged related differences and cardiovascular molecular calcification a 18-NaF PET/CT quantification of vascular calcification in the common carotid artery study [abstract]. J Nucl Med 2017;58(Suppl 1): 445.

83. Paydary K, Emamzadehfard S, Werner T, et al. Global assessment of cardiovascular NaF uptake is superior to FDG in the era of atherosclerosis imaging [abstract]. J Nucl Med 2017;58(Suppl 1): 977.

84. Emamzadehfard S, Raynor W, Acosta-Montenegro O, et al. Evolving role of FDG and NaF-PET/CT in early detection of peripheral artery diseases [abstract]. J Nucl Med 2017;58(Suppl 1):1019.

85. Shabahang C, Paydary K, Thomassen A, et al. Development of a novel quantitative approach for evaluation of cardiac calcification using 18F-NaF PET/CT [abstract]. J Nucl Med 2017;58(Suppl 1): 1183.

86. Al-Zaghal A, Seraj SM, Werner TJ, et al. Assessment of physiological intracranial calcification in healthy adults using 18F-NaF PET/CT. J Nucl Med 2018. https://doi.org/10.2967/jnumed.118.213678.

87. McKenney M, Territo P, Salavati A, et al. Assessment of 18F-NaF positron emission tomography imaging for early coronary artery calcification. FASEB J 2015;29:638.5.

88. Salavati A, Houshmand S, McKenney M, et al. Assessment of 18F-NaF PET/CT as a diagnostic tool for early detection of coronary artery calcification [abstract]. J Nucl Med 2015;56(Suppl3):460.

89. McKenney-Drake ML, Territo PR, Salavati A, et al. (18)F-NaF PET imaging of early coronary artery calcification. JACC Cardiovasc Imaging 2016;9:627–8.

90. Bural GG, Torigian DA, Chamroonrat W, et al. Quantitative assessment of the atherosclerotic burden of the aorta by combined FDG-PET and CT image analysis: a new concept. Nucl Med Biol 2006;33:1037–43.

91. Rogers IS, Nasir K, Figueroa AL, et al. Feasibility of FDG imaging of the coronary arteries: comparison between acute coronary syndrome and stable angina. JACC Cardiovasc Imaging 2010;3:388–97.

92. McKenney-Drake ML, Moghbel MC, Paydary K, et al. 18F-NaF and 18F-FDG as molecular probes in the evaluation of atherosclerosis. Eur J Nucl Med Mol Imaging 2018. https://doi.org/10.1007/s00259-018-4078-0.

93. Lee DL, Wamhoff BR, Katwa LC, et al. Increased endothelin-induced Ca2+ signaling, tyrosine phosphorylation, and coronary artery disease in diabetic dyslipidemic swine are prevented by atorvastatin. J Pharmacol Exp Ther 2003;306:132–40.

94. Majmudar MD, Yoo J, Keliher EJ, et al. Polymeric nanoparticle PET/MR imaging allows macrophage detection in atherosclerotic plaques. Circ Res 2013;112:755–61.

95. Nie X, Laforest R, Elvington A, et al. PET/MRI of hypoxic atherosclerosis using 64Cu-ATSM in a rabbit model. J Nucl Med 2016;57(12):2006–11.

96. Calcagno C, Lairez O, Hawkings J, et al. Combined PET/DCE-MRI in a rabbit model of atherosclerosis. JACC Cardiovasc Imaging 2018;11:291–301.

97. Ripa RS, Knudsen A, Hag AM, et al. Feasibility of simultaneous PET/MR of the carotid artery: first clinical experience and comparison to PET/CT. Am J Nucl Med Mol Imaging 2013;3:361–71.

98. Hyafil F, Schindler A, Sepp D, et al. High-risk plaque features can be detected in non-stenotic carotid plaques of patients with ischaemic stroke classified as cryptogenic using combined (18)F-FDG/MR imaging. Eur J Nucl Med Mol Imaging 2016;43:270–9.

99. Li X, Heber D, Rausch I, et al. Quantitative assessment of atherosclerotic plaques on (18)F-FDG PET/MRI: comparison with a PET/CT hybrid system. Eur J Nucl Med Mol Imaging 2016;43:1503–12.

100. Robson PM, Dweck MR, Trivieri MG, et al. Coronary artery PET/MR imaging: feasibility, limitations, and solutions. JACC Cardiovasc Imaging 2017;10(10 Pt A):1103–12.

101. Fernández-Ortiz A, Jiménez-Borreguero LJ, Peñalvo JL, et al. The progression and early detection of subclinical atherosclerosis (PESA) study: rationale and design. Am Heart J 2013;166:990–8.

102. Fernández-Friera L, Peñalvo JL, Fernández-Ortiz A, et al. Prevalence, vascular distribution, and multiterritorial extent of subclinical atherosclerosis in a middle-aged cohort: the PESA (progression of early subclinical atherosclerosis) study. Circulation 2015;131:2104–13.

103. Høilund-Carlsen PF, Hess S, Werner TJ, et al. Cancer metastasizes to the bone marrow and not to the bone: time for a paradigm shift! Eur J Nucl Med Mol Imaging 2018;45(6):893–7.

104. Alavi A, Werner TJ, Høilund-Carlsen PF, et al. Correction for partial volume effect is a must, not a luxury, to fully exploit the potential of quantitative PET imaging in clinical oncology. Mol Imaging Biol 2018;20(1):1–3.

PET-Based Imaging of Ischemic Heart Disease

Kevin Chen, MD[a], Edward J. Miller, MD, PhD[a], Mehran M. Sadeghi, MD[a,b,*]

KEYWORDS

- Coronary artery disease • Myocardial perfusion imaging • Coronary flow reserve
- Molecular imaging • Myocardial viability • PET/CTA hybrid imaging

KEY POINTS

- PET is an effective imaging modality for the diagnosis of coronary artery disease as well as assessing prognosis in patients with known disease.
- PET is the most sensitive modality to assess myocardial viability and provides an important tool in assessing the benefit of revascularization in patients with ischemic cardiomyopathy.
- Several exciting additions, including molecular imaging and introduction of new imaging tracers, are likely to increase the future use of cardiac PET.

INTRODUCTION

Ischemic heart disease is currently a leading cause of morbidity and mortality in the United States.[1] In recent decades, impressive advancements have been made in the diagnosis and treatment of coronary artery disease (CAD). Morbidity and mortality from CAD and its related complications, unfortunately, remain high in part due to the increasing prevalence of obesity and type 2 diabetes mellitus.

Nuclear cardiovascular imaging is a major player in the diagnosis and management of CAD. Myocardial perfusion imaging (MPI), in particular, fills an important role in its diagnosis, especially in patients of intermediate risk based on traditional risk factors as well as in assessment of risk for cardiac death or acute ischemic events in those with established disease. With its wide availability as well as a wealth of data backing its utility, single-photon emission CT (SPECT) has been the dominant MPI modality used for the diagnosis of CAD

as well as risk stratification of patients with known disease. PET-based MPI (**Figs. 1** and **2**), however, has increasing evidence to show its diagnostic utility and additive prognostic value. Furthermore, a recent position statement from American Society of Nuclear Cardiology/Society of Nuclear Medicine and Molecular Imaging advocates for PET MPI as the preferred stress imaging test for patients with known or suspected CAD who cannot undergo exercise stress testing.[2]

CURRENT CARDIAC PET RADIOTRACERS

Three perfusions tracers are potentially available for PET MPI: ^{82}Rb-rubidium chloride (^{82}Rb), ^{13}N-ammonia, and ^{15}O-water (**Table 1**),[3] and a few others are under development and evaluation (eg, ^{18}F-flupiridaz, 5-^{18}F-fluoropentyltriphenyl-phosphonium, and 6-^{18}F-fluorohexyltriphenyl-phosphonium).[4] Only ^{82}Rb and ^{13}N-ammonia are Food and Drug Administration-approved for clinical use in the United States. In addition to freedom

Disclosures: E.J. Miller: Consultant (GE, Inc; Bracco, Inc.); Grant Support (Bracco, Inc). M.M. Sadeghi: Consultant (Bracco Research USA).

Funding Sources: This work was supported by grants from NIH (R01-HL138567) and Department of Veterans Affairs (I0-BX001750).

[a] Section of Cardiovascular Medicine, Yale School of Medicine, 333 Cedar Street, New Haven, CT 06520, USA;
[b] Veterans Affairs Connecticut Healthcare System, 950 Campbell Avenue, West Haven, CT 06516, USA
* Corresponding author. Section of Cardiovascular Medicine, Yale School of Medicine, 333 Cedar Street, New Haven, CT 06520.
E-mail address: Mehran.Sadeghi@yale.edu

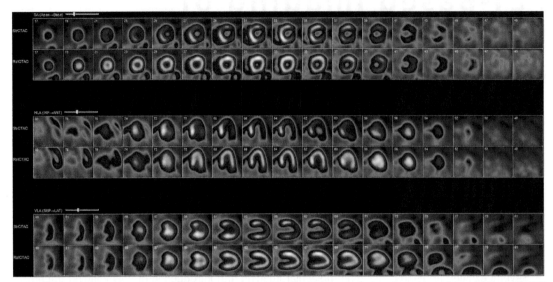

Fig. 1. ^{82}Rb PET MPI. Example of abnormal myocardial rest/stress perfusion imaging with rubidium-82 PET. Coregistered rest and stress images show a large reversible defect in the apex, apical anterior, and lateral walls consistent with ischemia. The patient had a drop in EF and evidence of transient ischemic dilatation of the left ventricle with stress. ANT, anterior; HLA, horizontal long axis; INF, inferior; LAT, lateral; RstCTAC, rest CT AC; SA, short axis; SEP, septal; StrCTAC, stress CT AC; VLA, vertical long axis.

from requiring an on-site cyclotron, ^{82}Rb PET MPI has significant advantages, including lower radiation exposure to patients compared with commonly used SPECT protocols and ^{13}N-ammonia PET, and is the most commonly used PET radiotracer for MPI. ^{13}N-ammonia may afford relatively higher sensitivity relative to ^{82}Rb due to its higher myocardial extraction (up to 80%) and trapping inside the cardiomyocytes after irreversible conversion to glutamine. Its main limitation is the requirement of an on-site cyclotron, which has precluded its widespread use. Novel benchtop ^{13}N-ammonia cyclotrons, however, have recently become commercially available, potentially allowing its more widespread application. The main advantage of ^{15}O-water is in providing near-perfect extraction fraction in comparison to myocardial blood flow (MBF).

DIAGNOSTIC ACCURACY AND PROGNOSTIC POTENTIAL

With increasing emphasis toward high-value care, a premium is placed on delivering quality care that adds value at lower costs. In cardiovascular medicine, this can be achieved with diagnostic testing delivering superior accuracy for obstructive CAD, one that stratifies patients into more-specific risk categories and correctly identifies those requiring further testing and/or interventions. PET MPI provides several advantages in this regard compared with conventional SPECT MPI.[5]

There is evidence supporting superior diagnostic accuracy of ^{82}Rb PET perfusion imaging compared with conventional SPECT MPI. Bateman and colleagues[6] showed that compared with SPECT MPI, PET MPI had a higher accuracy for identifying coronary stenosis severity of 70% (89% vs 79%; P = .03) and 50% (87% vs 71%; P = .003), with coronary angiography designated as the gold standard, and can better identify patients with multivessel disease compared with SPECT. Furthermore, PET imaging provided higher interpretive certainty, with more PET studies deemed definitively abnormal or normal versus SPECT, likely due to superior image quality. This study used risk-matched cohorts of patients for comparison and did not directly compare SPECT to PET. A meta-analysis by Mc Ardle and colleagues[7] showed similar findings even when attenuation correction (AC) and ECG gating were incorporated in SPECT MPI. With the introduction of newer PET/CT systems, studies have investigated the sensitivity and specificity in detecting coronary stenosis (compared with coronary angiography).[8–11] These data are summarized in **Fig. 3**. More recently, Danad and colleagues[12] reported on a prospective study comparing ^{15}O-water PET, ^{99m}Tc-tetrofosmin SPECT, and cardiac CT angiography (CCTA) for the diagnosis of hemodynamically significant CAD (defined as fractional flow reserve <0.8) in symptomatic patients with suspicion of coronary disease. PET had the highest diagnostic accuracy of 85% (95% CI,

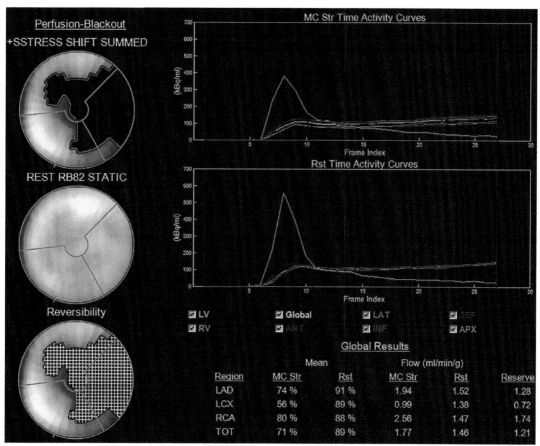

Fig. 2. Myocardial blood flows (MBFs) and flow reserve. MBF and Myocardial flow reserve (MFR) from patient in **Fig. 1.** Perfusion data on the 17-segment model on the left shows a large reversible defect mostly in the apex, apical anterior, and lateral walls. MFR is reduced in all 3 vascular territories, especially in that of the left circumflex. Global MFR is severely reduced (1.21). ANT, anterior; APX, apex; INF, inferior; LAD, left anterior descending; LAT, lateral; LCX, left circumflex; LV, left ventricle; MC, motion corrected; RCA, right coronary artery; Rst, rest; RV, right ventricle; SEPT, septal; SSTRESS, summed stress; Str, stress; TOT, total.

Table 1
Characteristics of PET radiotracers used for myocardial perfusion imaging

Characteristics	^{82}Rb-rubidium chloride	^{13}N-Ammonia	^{15}O-Water
Half-life	78 s	9.8 min	2.4 min
Extraction fraction[a]	~60%	~80%	~95%
Cyclotron on-site	No	Yes	Yes
Data acquisition	Dynamic, static, gated	Dynamic, static, gated	Dynamic
Scan duration	6 min	20 min	5 min
Dose (2-D PET)	40–60 mCi	15–25 mCi	40 mCi
Dose (3-D PET)	15–20 mCi 30–40 mCi 3D LSO	15 mCi	10 mCi
Interval between doses	10 min	30 min	7 min
Image interpretation	Yes	Yes	No
Image quality	Good	Excellent	N/A

Abbreviations: 2D, 2-dimensional; 3D, 3-dimensional; LSO, lutetium oxyorthosilicate.
 [a] Extraction fraction based on baseline MBF (~1 mL/g/min).
 Reproduced from Schelbert HR, Quercioli A, Dilsizian V. Cardiac PET imaging for the detection and monitoring of coronary artery disease and microvascular health. JACC Cardiovasc Imaging 2010;3(6):625; with permission.

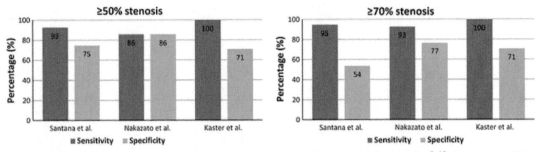

Fig. 3. Sensitivity and specificity of PET in detecting CAD. Results from 3 published studies[8–10] showing specificity and sensitivity in detecting coronary stenosis of ≥50% and ≥70% using automated-relative-quantification PET MPI with comparison to normal database. (*From* Slomka P, Berman DS, Alexanderson E, et al. The role of PET quantification in cardiovascular imaging. Clin Transl Imaging 2014;2(4):345; with permission.)

80%–90%) compared with CCTA (74%; 95% CI, 67%–79%; $P = .03$) and SPECT (77%; 95% CI, 71%–83%; $P = .02$).

Several reasons underlie the higher diagnostic accuracy of PET MPI. First, the use of coincidence detection imaging and high-count statistics in PET is associated with higher temporal and spatial resolution. Second, PET tracers have much higher photon energy (511 keV) compared with ^{99m}Tc-labeled SPECT tracers (140 keV), reducing Compton scatter and nonuniform attenuation. This is supplemented by the fact that ^{82}Rb has a short half-life, allowing higher doses, thus improving count statistics, with low radiation exposure. Third, CT-based AC is more routinely available in PET MPI. In a patient population where obesity is increasingly the norm, the problem of nonuniform attenuation due to excessive body habitus can cause significant artifacts, and AC can assist with improving specificity/image quality. Last, cardiac PET MPI provides additional diagnostic data, such as peak stress ejection fraction (EF), left ventricular (LV) EF reserve, and MBF quantification.

These additive characteristics enable PET MPI's use as a powerful prognostic tool. A normal PET MPI is associated with an exceedingly low risk (<1% annual rate of cardiac events) whereas an abnormal PET MPI result predicts higher rates of adverse cardiac events with risk proportional to the degree of abnormalities detected on perfusion imaging[13–15] (**Fig. 4**). Furthermore, given its higher image quality and accuracy, incremental changes in PET MPI may be easier to track throughout medical therapy for CAD. Sdringola and colleagues[16,17] showed that patients who received medical therapy along with lifestyle modifications exhibited improvement in outcomes as well as in previously detected perfusion imaging abnormalities in subsequent studies. In addition, higher-risk scans prior to initiation of therapy or worsening

abnormalities in subsequent studies were associated with worse prognosis.

QUANTIFICATION OF MYOCARDIAL FLOW AND FLOW RESERVE

Although most SPECT MPI studies are analyzed based on visual or at best semiquantitative assessment of relative perfusion defects, the use of dynamic acquisition sequences with PET provides a unique opportunity for absolute quantification of MBF. This affords several advantages to the clinician. Quantitative assessment of MBF and myocardial flow reserve (MFR), that is, as the ratio of MBF at hyperemic state and at rest, can provide information on total burden of both epicardial and microvascular disease. It can more reliably uncover multivessel disease, which, in cases of balanced ischemia, may be masked, leading to misdiagnosis of the extent of CAD.[3] Furthermore, there is evidence showing the added prognostic utility of absolute myocardial flow and reserve. Murthy and colleagues[18] demonstrated lower MFR correlated with higher cardiac mortality after adjusting for traditional cardiovascular risk factors, LVEF, and summed stress scores (SSSs) (hazard ratio [HR] 5.6 for lowest MFR vs highest MFR tertiles; 95% CI, 2.5–12.4; $P<.0001$; HR 3.4 for middle vs highest MFR tertiles; 95% CI, 1.5–7.7; $P = .003$). In addition, when MFR was incorporated into models assessing cardiac mortality risk with parameters such as LVEF and SSS, MFR reclassified 34% of patients at intermediate risk (1%–3% annual rate of death; net reclassification index: 0.484; 95% CI, 0.157–0.933). Ziadi and colleagues[19] similarly showed that lower myocardial flow and reserve in any class of SSS from relative perfusion imaging predicts higher risk of major cardiac adverse events (**Fig. 5**). Studies have also shown that in patients with cardiovascular risk factors, even with a normal PET/SPECT MPI or

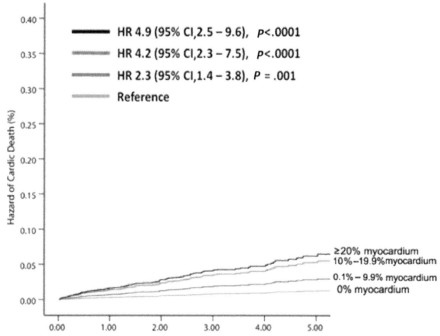

Fig. 4. Extent of perfusion abnormality and prognosis. Long-term follow-up data showing risk-adjusted hazard of cardiac death increases with increasing degree of perfusion abnormality (both ischemia and scar) on PET MPI. HR, hazard ratio. (*From* Dorbala S, Di Carli MF, Beanlands RS, et al. Prognostic value of stress myocardial perfusion positron emission tomography: results from a multicenter observational registry. J Am Coll Cardiol 2013;61(2):179; with permission.)

angiogram, an abnormal MBF/MFR independently identifies patients at risk of future cardiovascular events.[20,21] Information from MBF also allows the detection of early stages of CAD, prior to development of significant stenosis. As an example, changes in MFR in response to cold pressor testing, which is mediated by the sympathetic nervous system activation, allow the

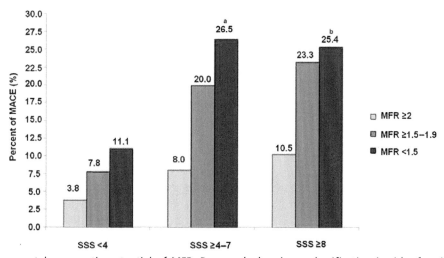

Fig. 5. Incremental prognostic potential of MFR. Bar graph showing reclassification in risk of major cardiac adverse events (MACE) with the incorporation of myocardial flow reserve (MFR) in each category of summed stress score (SSS) in PET MPI. [a] $P = .028$ for SSS $\geq$4 to 7 and MFR <1.5 versus MFR $\geq$2. [b] $P = .002$ for SSS $\geq$8 and MFR <1.5 versus MFR $\geq$2. (*From* Ziadi MC, Dekemp RA, Williams KA, et al. Impaired myocardial flow reserve on rubidium-82 positron emission tomography imaging predicts adverse outcomes in patients assessed for myocardial ischemia. J Am Coll Cardiol 2011;58(7):747; with permission.)

identification of patients who are at risk of CAD and the opportunity to consider early aggressive medical therapy. For example, Schindler and colleagues[22] showed that impaired MFR in response to cold pressor testing was associated with increased risk of adverse cardiac events. When incorporated into multivariate analysis along with other traditional cardiovascular risk factors, however, this relationship was no longer statistically significant (**Fig. 6**). Future prospective studies investigating this matter are warranted.

Certain groups of patients, including diabetics, women, and post–heart transplant patients, may benefit from PET MBF assessment. Diabetic patients are at heightened risk of CAD and associated adverse events but present a clinical challenge given their atypical and often asymptomatic presentations. Quinones and colleagues[23] found evidence of an inverse relationship between plasms glucose concentration and MFR, and it may be possible that PET-assessed MFR can identify diabetic individuals at the earliest stages of disease, even before onset of symptoms or changes in MPI or angiography. Women, particularly after menopause, are another group of challenging patients who may benefit from PET assessment of MFR. Taqueti and colleagues[24] showed in symptomatic patients referred for coronary angiography after PET MPI that women had more major adverse cardiac events than men despite less obstructive disease on angiography, and lower pretest clinical risk scores and rates of prior myocardial infarctions. Gender-related differences in MFR accounted for a majority of this increased risk for adverse events seen in women. Thus, MFR may be a useful tool for evaluation of female patients at risk for developing CAD and who may benefit from early aggressive medical

therapy. Further prospective studies are needed to confirm these findings. Another population that may benefit from MBF are post–heart transplant patients at risk for coronary vasculopathy.[25]

Although the data regarding the relative usefulness of MBF/MFR are encouraging, there must be cognizance of their potential pitfalls. Patient motion can introduce errors in the calculation of MBF and MFR due to count spillover from the LV blood pool into the myocardium and vice versa. Unlike traditional SPECT MPI, rotating raw projection images are not available, making detection of motion artifacts more difficult in PET. Furthermore, the timing of radiotracer injection relative to vasodilator administration is important and can be a source of error from failure to capture maximal hyperemia due to the relatively short half-lives of vasodilators used, most commonly now regadenoson.[26] The issue of reproducibility is important in assessment of MFB/MFR. Di Carli and colleagues[27] showed that this is particularly the case in patients with coronary lesions of intermediate severity because there was high variability in MBF of these patients. Without prior knowledge of coronary anatomy in these patients, it may be difficult to delineate between purely epicardial disease and microvascular dysfunction as the true cause of reduction in MBF/MFR. Finally, the calculation of MBF and MFR requires the estimation of arterial input function and a model to correct for nonlinear extraction of ^{82}Rb. Several methods currently are used to estimate these 2 entities, which can lead to variability of results.[28] In a retrospective study by Murthy and colleagues,[28] 3 methods, namely the region of interest, factor analysis and hybrid methods, were selected to estimate arterial input function in patients referred for PET stress testing. Rest

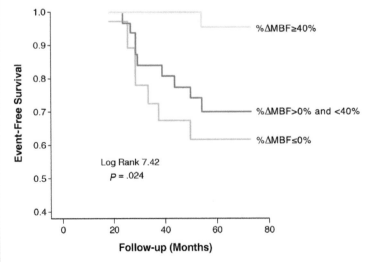

Fig. 6. Prognostic significance of coronary endothelial vasoreactivity. Kaplan-Meier curves showing event-free survival in patients with normal (group 1, ΔMBF ≥40%), impaired (group 2, ΔMBF >0% and <40%) and decreased (group 3, ΔMBF ≤0%) MBF to cold pressor testing. Patients with impaired and decreased MBF response to sympathetic stimulation were at increased risk of developing adverse cardiac events. (*From* Schindler TH, Schelbert HR, Quercioli A, et al. Cardiac PET imaging for the detection and monitoring of coronary artery disease and microvascular health. JACC Cardiovasc Imaging 2010;3(6):633; with permission.)

and stress MBF and MFR were calculated using each method, with 5 of the most common extraction models for ^{82}Rb. Results showed high variability in stress MBF in all 3 input function methods, particularly when using region of interest, but calculations of MFR showed significantly less variability. Consequently, there was high variability in the correlation between stress MBF and cardiac death but much less so in MFR regardless of input function used.[28] These data and potential pitfalls in MBF assessment are codified in a recent ASNC position statement.[29]

COST-EFFECTIVENESS WITH PET MYOCARDIAL PERFUSION IMAGING

Several studies in the past have shown potential for PET MPI to reduce costs.[30] One prospective study showed that although the cost of PET MPI was greater than SPECT MPI, this was more than offset by a decrease in downstream testing, namely coronary angiography and subsequent revascularization, along with additional costs of procedural complications, without a significant difference in clinical outcomes at 1 year. This was largely attributed to a much lower rate of false-positive testing in PET MPI versus its SPECT counterpart.[31] Other studies have shown the contrary, however. In a report from the Study of Myocardial Perfusion and Coronary Anatomy Imaging Roles in Coronary Artery Disease (SPARC trial), Hlatky and colleagues[32] showed that in patients undergoing PET, SPECT, and CT angiography (CTA) to evaluate for suspected CAD, those undergoing PET were associated with the highest costs and mortality at 2 years compared with SPECT or CTA. There is currently a lack of consensus in the optimal diagnostic protocol in MPI to maximize the cost/benefit ratio. Given the tremendous cost implications and the pressure to contain health care costs, however, future studies in this regard are needed.

ASSESSMENT OF MYOCARDIAL VIABILITY, ISCHEMIC MEMORY, AND INFLAMMATION

Besides the role it plays in MPI, PET has other applications in ischemic heart disease. In ischemic cardiomyopathy, ^{18}F-fluorodeoxyglucose (FDG) PET imaging is used to differentiate hibernating myocardium (the so-called viable myocardium) from scar, to identify the patients who might benefit from revascularization. Several recent clinical trials, however, have raised questions regarding the validity of this concept. In a substudy of the Surgical Treatment for Ischemic Heart Failure (STITCH) trial,[33] a randomized trial of medical therapy with or without coronary artery bypass grafting in patients with CAD and LV dysfunction, myocardial viability assessment did not identify patients with a differential survival benefit from coronary artery bypass grafting versus medical therapy alone.[34] The Positron Emission Tomography And Recovery Following Revascularization-1 (PARR-1) trial showed, in patients with ischemic cardiomyopathy with EF less than or equal to 35%, the amount of scar on FDG PET was a significant predictor of EF recovery after revascularization.[35] This did not translate, however, into positive outcomes in the PARR-2 trial, which failed to show reduced adverse cardiac events when these patients were randomized to a PET-guided management strategy compared with standard care at 1 year follow-up. Post hoc analysis of the data showed that patients who adhered to PET-guided recommendations benefited significantly,[36] supporting a potential role for viability assessment in this setting, which requires further investigation. Other data suggest that PET may identify myocardium at risk of adverse remodeling and cardiomyopathy after myocardial infarction. In a study by Rischpler and colleagues,[37] significant myocardial FDG uptake 5 days after an ST elevation myocardial infarction was associated with markers of poor cardiac function, such as reduction EF and increases in end-diastolic volume and end-systolic volume assessed by MR imaging 6 months after MI. Finally, another potential application of PET is to identify myocardium that recently experienced ischemia, a phenomenon called ischemic memory. This is due to metabolic changes of ischemic myocardium, resulting in decreased metabolism of fatty acids, its usual energy source, and increased metabolism of glucose.[38]

PET/CT ANGIOGRAPHY HYBRID IMAGING

Hybrid PET/CTA imaging combines anatomic information from CTA with myocardial perfusion data obtained from PET and may provide complementary data.[39] In a prospective study involving 107 patients with intermediate probability of CAD, Kajander and colleagues[40] showed hybrid quantitative PET with CTA had significantly greater diagnostic accuracy for detecting significant CAD (defined by ≥50% vessel stenosis) than either alone. Gaemperli and colleagues[41] and Danad and colleagues[12] showed similar results purporting the diagnostic accuracy in PET/CTA hybrid imaging. Currently, the use of PET/CTA hybrid imaging is rare, and several limitations, including cost and increased exposure to radiation, need to be addressed. As an alternative, Maaniitty and colleagues[42] proposed imaging with PET MPI only after significant CAD is identified on CTA, because patients with normal CTA have very low rates of adverse outcomes.

FUTURE DIRECTIONS

Exciting new developments are currently under way for PET-based imaging for ischemic heart disease. Among these is the development ^{18}F-labeled flow tracers, for example, ^{18}F-flurpiridaz. Potential advantages of ^{18}F-flurpiridaz include a higher extraction fraction compared with [82]Rb, allowing higher sensitivity in detecting perfusion defects as well as better assessment of MBF/MFR.[43–45] The longer half-life of ^{18}F also makes it compatible with exercise stress testing. In terms of logistics, the longer half-life of ^{18}F necessitates only a regional cyclotron for production rather than an onsite cyclotron. Preliminary data from the first phase 3 trial showed ^{18}F-flurpiridaz PET MPI was statistically superior to ^{99m}Tc-tetrofosmin or sestamibi SPECT MPI in sensitivity of CAD detection, defined by gold standard coronary angiography as stenosis greater than 50%, or documentation of prior myocardial infarction (71.9% vs 53.7%; P<.001). It failed to achieve its second primary outcome, however, noninferiority in specificity, compared with SPECT MPI (72.6% vs 82.6%; P = .9450). Flurpiridaz MPI also exposed patients to less radiation compared with SPECT (6.1 mSv ± 0.4 mSv vs 13.4 mSv ± 3.2 mSv; P<.01) and had higher diagnostic certainty (P<.001) and superior image quality (P<.001). In subgroup analysis, sensitivity of ^{18}F-flurpiridaz PET MPI was superior in obese patients (body mass index >30) and female patients.[46] Currently a second phase III trial is under way (ClinicalTrials.gov identifier: NCT03354273).

Another exciting development is the tremendous potential of PET-based molecular imaging in ischemic heart disease. Emerging molecular imaging techniques seek to image biological features of atherosclerotic lesions (eg, inflammation and microcalcification), which predispose coronary plaques to rupture. Rudd and colleagues[47] showed a differential uptake of FDG in carotid artery atherosclerotic plaques in symptomatic and asymptomatic patients. Since this landmark study, multiple studies have shown an association between vascular FDG uptake and cardiovascular risk factors, such as diabetes[48] and metabolic syndrome,[49] as well as Framingham risk score.[50] These observations have been attributed to the ability of FDG PET to detect vascular inflammation.[51,52] FDG PET imaging of vascular inflammation suffers from poor specificity, however, because any metabolically active tissue using primarily glucose can take up FDG. Due to the small size of coronary arteries, cardiac motion, and myocardial uptake of the tracer, FDG PET imaging of coronary arteries remains challenging, and issues related to quantification methodology and optimal preparation of subjects prior to imaging remain to be fully addressed.[53] Several alternative PET-based strategies to imaging vascular inflammation are emerging, which may detect cardiac and coronary inflammation in ischemic heart disease.[54–57] Given the potential association of microcalcification with plaque vulnerability, ^{18}F-sodium fluoride (NaF) PET may be of value in this setting. Joshi and colleagues[58] reported that, in patients with myocardial infarction, NaF PET can identify culprit coronary lesions. Further studies are required to assess the ability of this agent in risk stratification and management of patients with CAD.

In the coming years, it is expected that PET-based imaging of ischemic heart disease will increase in prevalence. Currently, [82]Rb is the most widely used PET tracer for assessment of CAD, and although there are known limitations to the use of this radiotracer, evidence of the high diagnostic accuracy and the added prognostic potential of [82]Rb PET MPI make it an attractive alternative to its SPECT counterpart, especially in certain groups of patients, such as those with obesity. Furthermore, with exciting developments in new PET radiotracers, advances in molecular imaging, and progress in hybrid imaging with CT or MR imaging, PET based imaging will continue to play a prominent role in evaluation of ischemic heart disease.

CLINICAL PEARLS FOR THE REFERRING PROVIDER

- PET MPI is a powerful tool in the diagnosis of CAD and assessing prognosis for those with known disease. There is evidence showing its superior diagnostic and prognostic potential compared with conventional SPECT MPI in patients with coronary disease.
- Information from MBFs allows early detection of coronary disease in certain groups of patients at high risk of CAD, such as diabetics and postmenopausal women.
- PET MPI can produce higher image quality and interpretive certainty compared with SPECT MPI, and studies are done in less time with less radiation exposure to patients.
- Due to short half-life of the tracer, [82]Rb PET MPI studies cannot be done with exercise.

- Patients referred for MPI and unable to exercise should be considered for PET. This is especially true for obese patients whose body habitus may be problematic with other MPI modalities.
- PET is also useful for assessment of myocardial viability in patients with ischemic cardiomyopathy.
- Exciting opportunities are arising in molecular imaging, which may increase the use of PET imaging for ischemic heart disease in the future.

REFERENCES

1. Murphy SL, Xu J, Kochanek KD, et al. Deaths: final data for 2015. Natl Vital Stat Rep 2017;66(6):1–75.
2. Bateman TM, Dilsizian V, Beanlands RS, et al. American Society of Nuclear Cardiology and Society of Nuclear Medicine and molecular imaging joint position statement on the clinical indications for myocardial perfusion PET. J Nucl Med 2016;57(10):1654–6.
3. Schindler TH, Schelbert HR, Quercioli A, et al. Cardiac PET imaging for the detection and monitoring of coronary artery disease and microvascular health. JACC Cardiovasc Imaging 2010;3(6):623–40.
4. Brunken RC. Promising new 18F-labeled tracers for PET myocardial perfusion imaging. J Nucl Med 2015;56(10):1478–9.
5. Radiation dose to patients from cardiac diagnostic imaging. Circulation 2007;116(11):1290–305.
6. Bateman TM, Heller GV, McGhie AI, et al. Diagnostic accuracy of rest/stress ECG-gated Rb-82 myocardial perfusion PET: comparison with ECG-gated Tc-99m sestamibi SPECT. J Nucl Cardiol 2006;13(1):24–33.
7. Mc Ardle BA, Dowsley TF, deKemp RA, et al. Does rubidium-82 PET have superior accuracy to SPECT perfusion imaging for the diagnosis of obstructive coronary disease?: a systematic review and meta-analysis. J Am Coll Cardiol 2012;60(18):1828–37.
8. Kaster T, Mylonas I, Renaud JM, et al. Accuracy of low-dose rubidium-82 myocardial perfusion imaging for detection of coronary artery disease using 3D PET and normal database interpretation. J Nucl Cardiol 2012;19(6):1135–45.
9. Santana CA, Folks RD, Garcia EV, et al. Quantitative (82)Rb PET/CT: development and validation of myocardial perfusion database. J Nucl Med 2007;48(7):1122–8.
10. Nakazato R, Berman DS, Dey D, et al. Automated quantitative Rb-82 3D PET/CT myocardial perfusion imaging: normal limits and correlation with invasive coronary angiography. J Nucl Cardiol 2012;19(2):265–76.
11. Slomka P, Berman DS, Alexanderson E, et al. The role of PET quantification in cardiovascular imaging. Clin Transl Imaging 2014;2(4):343–58.
12. Danad I, Raijmakers PG, Driessen RS, et al. Comparison of coronary CT angiography, SPECT, PET, and hybrid imaging for diagnosis of ischemic heart disease determined by fractional flow reserve. JAMA Cardiol 2017;2(10):1100–7.
13. Dorbala S, Di Carli MF, Beanlands RS, et al. Prognostic value of stress myocardial perfusion positron emission tomography: results from a multicenter observational registry. J Am Coll Cardiol 2013;61(2):176–84.
14. Dorbala S, Hachamovitch R, Curillova Z, et al. Incremental prognostic value of gated Rb-82 positron emission tomography myocardial perfusion imaging over clinical variables and rest LVEF. JACC Cardiovasc Imaging 2009;2(7):846–54.
15. Yoshinaga K, Chow BJ, Williams K, et al. What is the prognostic value of myocardial perfusion imaging using rubidium-82 positron emission tomography? J Am Coll Cardiol 2006;48(5):1029–39.
16. Sdringola S, Nakagawa K, Nakagawa Y, et al. Combined intense lifestyle and pharmacologic lipid treatment further reduce coronary events and myocardial perfusion abnormalities compared with usual-care cholesterol-lowering drugs in coronary artery disease. J Am Coll Cardiol 2003;41(2):263–72.
17. Sdringola S, Gould KL, Zamarka LG, et al. A 6 month randomized, double blind, placebo controlled, multicenter trial of high dose atorvastatin on myocardial perfusion abnormalities by positron emission tomography in coronary artery disease. Am Heart J 2008;155(2):245–53.
18. Murthy VL, Naya M, Foster CR, et al. Improved cardiac risk assessment with noninvasive measures of coronary flow reserve. Circulation 2011;124(20):2215–24.
19. Ziadi MC, Dekemp RA, Williams KA, et al. Impaired myocardial flow reserve on rubidium-82 positron emission tomography imaging predicts adverse outcomes in patients assessed for myocardial ischemia. J Am Coll Cardiol 2011;58(7):740–8.
20. Herzog BA, Husmann L, Valenta I, et al. Long-term prognostic value of 13N-ammonia myocardial perfusion positron emission tomography added value of coronary flow reserve. J Am Coll Cardiol 2009;54(2):150–6.
21. Taqueti VR, Hachamovitch R, Murthy VL, et al. Global coronary flow reserve is associated with adverse cardiovascular events independently of luminal angiographic severity and modifies the effect of early revascularization. Circulation 2015;131(1):19–27.
22. Schindler TH, Nitzsche EU, Schelbert HR, et al. Positron emission tomography-measured abnormal responses of myocardial blood flow to sympathetic stimulation are associated with the risk of developing cardiovascular events. J Am Coll Cardiol 2005;45(9):1505–12.

23. Quinones MJ, Hernandez-Pampaloni M, Schelbert H, et al. Coronary vasomotor abnormalities in insulin-resistant individuals. Ann Intern Med 2004;140(9):700–8.

24. Taqueti VR, Shaw LJ, Cook NR, et al. Excess cardiovascular risk in women relative to men referred for coronary angiography is associated with severely impaired coronary flow reserve, not obstructive disease. Circulation 2017;135(6):566–77.

25. Chih S, Chong AY, Erthal F, et al. PET assessment of epicardial intimal disease and microvascular dysfunction in cardiac allograft vasculopathy. J Am Coll Cardiol 2018;71(13):1444–56.

26. Johnson NP, Gould KL. Regadenoson versus dipyridamole hyperemia for cardiac PET imaging. JACC Cardiovasc Imaging 2015;8(4):438–47.

27. Di Carli M, Czernin J, Hoh CK, et al. Relation among stenosis severity, myocardial blood flow, and flow reserve in patients with coronary artery disease. Circulation 1995;91(7):1944–51.

28. Murthy VL, Lee BC, Sitek A, et al. Comparison and prognostic validation of multiple methods of quantification of myocardial blood flow with 82Rb PET. J Nucl Med 2014;55(12):1952–8.

29. Murthy VL, Bateman TM, Beanlands RS, et al. Clinical quantification of myocardial blood flow using PET: joint position paper of the SNMMI cardiovascular council and the ASNC. J Nucl Cardiol 2018;25(1):269–97.

30. Patterson RE, Eisner RL, Horowitz SF. Comparison of cost-effectiveness and utility of exercise ECG, single photon emission computed tomography, positron emission tomography, and coronary angiography for diagnosis of coronary artery disease. Circulation 1995;91(1):54–65.

31. Merhige ME, Breen WJ, Shelton V, et al. Impact of myocardial perfusion imaging with PET and (82)Rb on downstream invasive procedure utilization, costs, and outcomes in coronary disease management. J Nucl Med 2007;48(7):1069–76.

32. Hlatky MA, Shilane D, Hachamovitch R, et al. Economic outcomes in the study of myocardial perfusion and coronary anatomy imaging roles in coronary artery disease registry: the SPARC Study. J Am Coll Cardiol 2014;63(10):1002–8.

33. Velazquez EJ, Lee KL, Deja MA, et al. Coronary-artery bypass surgery in patients with left ventricular dysfunction. N Engl J Med 2011;364(17):1607–16.

34. Bonow RO, Maurer G, Lee KL, et al. Myocardial viability and survival in ischemic left ventricular dysfunction. N Engl J Med 2011;364(17):1617–25.

35. Beanlands RS, Ruddy TD, deKemp RA, et al. Positron emission tomography and recovery following revascularization (PARR-1): the importance of scar and the development of a prediction rule for the degree of recovery of left ventricular function. J Am Coll Cardiol 2002;40(10):1735–43.

36. Beanlands RS, Nichol G, Huszti E, et al. F-18-fluoro-deoxyglucose positron emission tomography imaging-assisted management of patients with severe left ventricular dysfunction and suspected coronary disease: a randomized, controlled trial (PARR-2). J Am Coll Cardiol 2007;50(20):2002–12.

37. Rischpler C, Dirschinger RJ, Nekolla SG, et al. Prospective evaluation of 18F-fluorodeoxyglucose uptake in postischemic myocardium by simultaneous positron emission tomography/magnetic resonance imaging as a prognostic marker of functional outcome. Circ Cardiovasc Imaging 2016;9(4):e004316.

38. Jain D, He ZX, Lele V, et al. Direct myocardial ischemia imaging: a new cardiovascular nuclear imaging paradigm. Clin Cardiol 2015;38(2):124–30.

39. Gaemperli O, Bengel FM, Kaufmann PA. Cardiac hybrid imaging. Eur Heart J 2011;32(17):2100–8.

40. Kajander S, Joutsiniemi E, Saraste M, et al. Cardiac positron emission tomography/computed tomography imaging accurately detects anatomically and functionally significant coronary artery disease. Circulation 2010;122(6):603–13.

41. Gaemperli O, Saraste A, Knuuti J. Cardiac hybrid imaging. Eur Heart J Cardiovasc Imaging 2012;13(1):51–60.

42. Maaniitty T, Stenstrom I, Bax JJ, et al. Prognostic value of coronary CT angiography with selective PET perfusion imaging in coronary artery disease. JACC Cardiovasc Imaging 2017;10(11):1361–70.

43. Huisman MC, Higuchi T, Reder S, et al. Initial characterization of an 18F-labeled myocardial perfusion tracer. J Nucl Med 2008;49(4):630–6.

44. Maddahi J. Properties of an ideal PET perfusion tracer: new PET tracer cases and data. J Nucl Cardiol 2012;19(Suppl 1):S30–7.

45. Yalamanchili P, Wexler E, Hayes M, et al. Mechanism of uptake and retention of F-18 BMS-747158-02 in cardiomyocytes: a novel PET myocardial imaging agent. J Nucl Cardiol 2007;14(6):782–8.

46. Abstracts of original contributions ASNC2015 the 20th annual scientific session of the American Society of Nuclear Cardiology. J Nucl Cardiol 2015;22(4):744–81.

47. Rudd JH, Warburton EA, Fryer TD, et al. Imaging atherosclerotic plaque inflammation with [18F]-fluorodeoxyglucose positron emission tomography. Circulation 2002;105(23):2708–11.

48. Bucerius J, Mani V, Moncrieff C, et al. Impact of noninsulin-dependent type 2 diabetes on carotid wall 18F-fluorodeoxyglucose positron emission tomography uptake. J Am Coll Cardiol 2012;59(23):2080–8.

49. Tahara N, Kai H, Yamagishi S, et al. Vascular inflammation evaluated by [18F]-fluorodeoxyglucose positron emission tomography is associated with the

metabolic syndrome. J Am Coll Cardiol 2007;49(14): 1533–9.

50. Noh TS, Moon SH, Cho YS, et al. Relation of carotid artery 18F-FDG uptake to C-reactive protein and Framingham risk score in a large cohort of asymptomatic adults. J Nucl Med 2013;54(12): 2070–6.

51. Myers KS, Rudd JH, Hailman EP, et al. Correlation between arterial FDG uptake and biomarkers in peripheral artery disease. JACC Cardiovasc Imaging 2012;5(1):38–45.

52. Menezes LJ, Kotze CW, Agu O, et al. Investigating vulnerable atheroma using combined (18)F-FDG PET/CT angiography of carotid plaque with immunohistochemical validation. J Nucl Med 2011;52(11): 1698–703.

53. Sadeghi MM. 18)F-FDG PET and vascular inflammation: time to refine the paradigm? J Nucl Cardiol 2015;22(2):319–24.

54. Tavakoli S, Vashist A, Sadeghi MM. Molecular imaging of plaque vulnerability. J Nucl Cardiol 2014; 21(6):1112–28.

55. Tarkin JM, Dweck MR, Evans NR, et al. Imaging atherosclerosis. Circ Res 2016;118(4):750–69.

56. Derlin T, Sedding DG, Dutzmann J, et al. Imaging of chemokine receptor CXCR4 expression in culprit and nonculprit coronary atherosclerotic plaque using motion-corrected [(68)Ga]pentixafor PET/CT. Eur J Nucl Med Mol Imaging 2018; 45(11):1934–44.

57. Tarkin JM, Joshi FR, Evans NR, et al. Detection of atherosclerotic inflammation by (68)Ga-DOTATATE PET compared to [(18)F]FDG PET imaging. J Am Coll Cardiol 2017;69(14):1774–91.

58. Joshi NV, Vesey AT, Williams MC, et al. 18F-fluoride positron emission tomography for identification of ruptured and high-risk coronary atherosclerotic plaques: a prospective clinical trial. Lancet 2014; 383(9918):705–13.

PET/CT Evaluation of Cardiac Sarcoidosis

John P. Bois, MD[a],*, Daniele Muser, MD[b,1], Panithaya Chareonthaitawee, MD[a]

KEYWORDS

• Cardiac sarcoidosis • Positron emission tomography • Fluorine-18 deoxyglucose

KEY POINTS

• Sarcoidosis can involve the heart at with resultant significant morbidity and mortality.
• PET/CT is the most accurate method by which to diagnose cardiac sarcoidosis.
• Patient preparation prior to the PET/CT cardiac sarcoid study is critical to ensure diagnostic images are obtained.
• PET/CT detection of both active inflammation and scar has diagnostic, prognostic, and therapeutic importance.
• Ongoing areas of research include the use of PET to quantify the extent of myocardial inflammation and the discrepancies in myocardial blood flow in the cardiac sarcoidosis population.

INTRODUCTION

The increasing implementation of advanced cardiovascular imaging in the form of cardiac PET/CT has had a significant impact on the management of cardiac sarcoidosis (CS), one that continues to evolve. Sarcoidosis is characterized histologically by the presence of noncaseating granulomas, with a predilection for the pulmonary system but with the ability to involve nearly every organ. Although the development of sarcoidosis is believed the sequelae of an exaggerated immune or inflammatory response to an inciting infectious or environmental trigger, the specific etiology of this disease remains elusive. The exact prevalence of sarcoidosis is unknown but tends to be highest in women ages 25 years to 44 years (100 in 100,000) and in African Americans.[1,2] There is also a geographic predilection for the development of sarcoidosis, with some regions within the United States reporting rates as high as 330 in 100,000 patients.[2] The course of the disease is variable, with approximately two-thirds of patients experiencing spontaneous remission and the remaining one-third developing either a stable or progressive course.[3]

The rate of cardiac involvement by sarcoidosis, otherwise termed CS, is variable and ranges from 20% to 75%.[4,5] Furthermore, CS accounts for one-fourth of sarcoid-related mortality in the United States and upward of 85% of death attributed to sarcoidosis in the Japanese population.[4,6] The high rate of involvement of the cardiovascular system by sarcoidosis coupled with the potential lethal outcomes has rendered accurate and timely diagnosis of this disease entity as imperative to patient care. Unfortunately, the prompt recognition of CS itself may be elusive, with both traditional imaging techniques as well as invasive endomyocardial biopsies often providing a low diagnostic yield.[6] Consequently, there have been focused efforts to enhance or to develop noninvasive imaging techniques that not only detect CS but also potentially provide therapeutic and prognostic information for the treating clinician. Cardiac PET/CT has emerged as a leading modality

Conflict of Interest: The authors have no disclosures.
[a] Department of Cardiovascular Diseases, Mayo Clinic, 200 First Street Southwest, Rochester, MN 55905, USA;
[b] Cardiovascular Division, Hospital of The University of Pennsylvania, Philadelphia, PA, USA
[1] Present address: Via Pallanza 101, Udine 33100, Italy.
* Corresponding author.
E-mail address: Bois.John@mayo.edu

PET Clin 14 (2019) 223–232
https://doi.org/10.1016/j.cpet.2018.12.004
1556-8598/19/© 2018 Elsevier Inc. All rights reserved.

by which to begin to address these issues for the CS patient population.

INDICATIONS FOR CARDIAC PET/CT FOR CARDIAC SARCOIDOSIS

The limited size of investigational studies involving the CS population and the lack of available prospective data have resulted in the inability to formulate evidence-based guidelines to determine which patients warrant PET/CT imaging for the assessment of CS.[7,8] The traditional diagnostic guideline for the detection of CS, as outlined by the Japanese Ministry of Health, Labour and Welfare, did not include PET/CT imaging.[6] The more contemporary guidelines, as proposed by the Heart Rhythm Society in 2014 and the revised Japanese Society of Cardiac Sarcoidosis in 2017, did include PET/CT as a component of the diagnostic algorithm.[9,10] The surmised improved diagnostic capabilities of the Heart Rhythm Society and the revised Japanese Society of Sarcoidosis criteria due to the inclusion of PET/CT have yet to be systematically tested.

Given the absence of evidence-based guidelines, Chareonthaitawee and colleagues[8] have issued a joint expert consensus document on behalf of the Society of Nuclear Medicine and Molecular Imaging (SNMMI) and the American Society of Nuclear Cardiology (ASNC), which outlines the following 4 patient scenarios for which cardiac PET/CT for the assessment of CS could be considered:

- Histologic evidence of extra CS *and* 1 or more abnormal screening results for CS (ECG demonstrating completed left and/or right bundle branch block, unexplained Q waves in 2 or more ECG leads, echocardiographic evidence of regional wall motion abnormalities and/or aneurysms, basal septal thinning or depressed left ventricular ejection fraction (<50%), ventricular tachycardia, MR imaging evidence of midmyocardial inflammation, and, lastly, unexplained palpitations or syncope)
- New-onset sustained second-degree or third-degree atrioventricular block *and* age less than 60 years old
- Idiopathic sustained ventricular tachycardia
- Serial studies to assess response to treatment

As cardiac PET/CT is further refined, standardized, and utilized and as awareness of CS expands, future evidenced-based guidelines may become available. Until that juncture, however, the aforementioned 4 patient scenarios as outlined by experts in the field provide a useful tool for clinicians in determining when to order a cardiac PET/CT for the evaluation of CS.

PATIENT PREPARATION FOR CARDIAC PET/CT FOR CARDIAC SARCOIDOSIS

Optimal patient preparation is essential when using fluorine-18 deoxyglucose (^{18}F-FDG) PET/CT to evaluate for CS. The predilection for ^{18}F-FDG accumulation within inflamed tissues, in particular macrophages, is the pathophysiologic underpinning of ^{18}F-FDG PET/CT CS imaging. It is imperative, therefore, that physiologic myocardial uptake of ^{18}F-FDG be suppressed to identify areas of pathologic involvement in a manner tht is both accurate and reproducible.[11] Consequently, several methods have been developed to achieve suppression of physiologic ^{18}F-FDG uptake.

Cardiac myocyte metabolism is a dynamic and complex process that involves selective uses of variable fuel sources, including free fatty acids, glucose, and ketones.[12] Which substrate is preferentially used is determined by a combination of physiologic variables, including substrate availability, myocardial blood flow (MBF), and serum insulin concentration.[13] In the postprandial state, increased serum insulin levels result in glucose transporter 1 and glucose transporter 2 upregulation, resulting in increased myocyte glucose uptake.[14] One method by which to avoid physiologic myocyte uptake is instituting a prolonged fast. During the fasting state, lipids in lieu of glucose become the preferred myocyte substrate and this is particularly the case with prolonged fasting of upward of 18 hours.[15] Prior studies have demonstrated that the success rates of fasting protocols in suppressing physiologic ^{18}F-FDG range from 62% to 90% (**Fig. 1**).[16–19] Unfortunately, prolonged fasting often proves laborious, and the lack of patient compliance is a concern.[20,21] Furthermore, hypoglycemia potentially develops with the use of this technique.[16]

A potential alternative to the prolonged fast is the implementation of a diet consisting of high fat and low carbohydrates. Studies have demonstrated that this technique may be superior to fasting alone.[22] Concern again arises, however, regarding the ability of patients to adhere to such dietary recommendations due to potential religious or cultural beliefs or due to an inability to tolerate such a diet. Another potential means by which to increase serum free fatty acid levels is via the use of unfractionated heparin (typically administered dose is 50 U/kg approximately 15 minutes prior to ^{18}F-FDG administration), which stimulates lipolysis.[16,23,24] A prior investigation of healthy volunteers demonstrated that unfractionated heparin could successfully increase free fatty acid levels without prolonging the partial thromboplastin time.[25] Subsequent evaluations of the

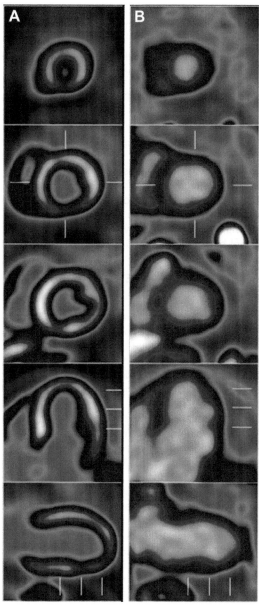

Fig. 1. ^{18}F-FDG and N-13 ammonia PET/CT for CS. No perfusion defects are present on N-13 ammonia imaging (*A*). ^{18}F-FDG is present only in the blood pool with no myocardial uptake, consistent with effective suppression of physiologic myocardial glucose and a normal study (*B*). *Panel A* is the perfusion panel as listed. From top to bottom is apex, mid, and base then horizontal and vertical long axis. *Panel B* is FDG panel as listed and from top to bottom is apex, mid, and base then horizontal and vertical long axis.

efficacy of unfractionated heparin, however, have reported conflicting results rendering its utilization uncertain.[16,17,24]

Given the myriad options for patient preparation and the potential confusion that may subsequently

result, there has been a call to standardize protocols and to develop preparation guidelines.[11] As a result, both the SNMMI and the ASNC have officially recommended at least 2 high-fat (>35 g) and low-carbohydrate (<3 g) meals a day prior to the anticipated ^{18}F-FDG PET/CT followed by a fast of 4 hours to 12 hours prior to the study, with an alternative a prolonged fast of 18 hours.[26] To implement such guidelines, patient education prior to the study is imperative, with materials to facilitate such a discussion having been previously published.[27]

Regardless of the exact methodology used to prepare patients for the study, nuclear physicians should be aware of 2 specific patient populations that provide unique challenges. The first is diabetic patients for whom an optimal dietary preparation has not been identified. Insulin-dependent diabetic patients should continue basal insulin with minimization of rapid-acting insulin. If needed, a sliding scale may be implemented the day before but not the day of the study.[8] For non–insulin-dependent patients, oral hypoglycemic agents should be avoided during periods of prescribed fasting.[8]

Unfortunately, despite extensive efforts to prohibit physiologic myocardial ^{18}F-FDG uptake, approximately 30% of potential CS patients have an inconclusive scan, resulting in patient and provider frustration, nondiagnostic exposure to radiation, and financial loss (**Fig. 2**).[11,16,20,28–30] Consequently, the development of a radiotracer that does not demonstrate physiologic myocardial uptake and does not require dietary preparation would be of great potential benefit to the PET/CT assessment of the CS population. Gallium-68 (^{68}Ga) DOTATAE, a radiotracer targeted toward somatostatin receptors, is a potential alternative to ^{18}F-FDG in imaging in the CS patient. Initially developed to assess neuroendocrine tumors,[31] ^{68}Ga-DOTATAE also targets activated macrophages and multinucleated cells, which express somatostatin receptors, but does not target normal myocardial tissue, which lacks such receptors.[32] Therefore, ^{68}Ga-DOTATAE potentially obviates patient preparation protocols and could limit the incidence of uninterpretable scans. An initial feasibility study[33] followed by a small trial of 19 patients demonstrated promising results,[32] with further investigations anticipated.

PERFORMANCE OF PET/CT FOR ASSESSMENT OF CARDIAC SARCOIDOSIS

PET/CT assessment of CS is composed of 2 resting images—one to assess myocardial perfusion and the second to assess myocardial

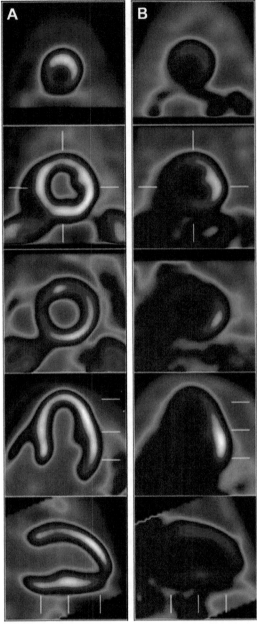

Fig. 2. ^{18}F-FDG and N-13 ammonia PET/CT for CS. No perfusion defects are present on N-13 ammonia imaging (*A*). ^{18}F-FDG images demonstrated diffuse uptake throughout the entire myocardium with areas of focal on diffuse uptake. These findings are nonspecific and are likely secondary to ineffective suppression of physiologic myocardial glucose uptake (*B*). *Panel A* is the perfusion panel as listed. From top to bottom is apex, mid, and base then horizontal and vertical long axis. *Panel B* is FDG panel as listed and from top to bottom is apex, mid, and base then horizontal and vertical long axis.

inflammation. A gated perfusion study is performed first utilizing either N-13 ammonia or rubidium-82. Gating is critical because it allows for assessment of left ventricular ejection fraction

as well as regional wall motion abnormalities. After the perfusion study, the inflammatory assessment scan is performed, with ^{18}F-FDG the most common radiotracer used. Approximately a 60-minute to 90-minute uptake period for ^{18}F-FDG is required, followed by a 10-minute to 30-minute nongated acquisition.[34] The field of view for the inflammation acquisition scan may be focused on the heart alone or may be extended to include base of the skill to the upper thigh. The latter is typically recommended if clinical suspicion of extracardiac sarcoid exists or a recent whole-body investigation has not been completed, because the detection of extracardiac disease may have diagnostic and prognostic implications as well as potentially providing targets for subsequent biopsy attempts (**Fig. 3**).[8]

INTERPRETATION OF PET/CT CARDIAC SARCOIDOSIS STUDIES

As recommended with traditional PET/CT perfusion imaging, a systematic approach to image interpretation is considered optimal practice. Image interpretation begins with quality-control assessment, including determination of proper coregistration between the transmission (CT) and emission (PET) scans.[34] Misalignment between the 2 scans can occur for multiple reasons, including voluntary and involuntary patient movement.[35] Prior studies have reported that upward of 40% of cardiac PET/CT scans demonstrate false-positive perfusion defects secondary to misregistration.[36] Careful attention should be made for anterior and lateral myocardial perfusion defects because these territories are most prone to misalignment artifacts between the transmission and emission images. Another critical step in the quality-control process is to ensure that there is adequate suppression of physiologic myocardial ^{18}F-FDG uptake. Adequate suppression is considered to be no visible uptake or at least uptake lower than the blood pool.[26]

After determination of the quality of the study, the authors' typical practice is to assess left ventricular size and ejection fraction. Subsequently, a simultaneous qualitative assessment is performed of both the myocardial perfusion and the inflammatory images.[37,38] A resting myocardial perfusion defect could be attributed to microvascular compression from inflammation or may be due to scar. If concurrent ^{18}F-FDG is noted in the same territory, then the perfusion defect is likely secondary to inflammation (**Fig. 4**). If ^{18}F-FDG uptake is lacking in this territory and if a regional wall motion abnormality exits, then scar is favored (**Fig. 5**). Myocardial inflammation secondary to

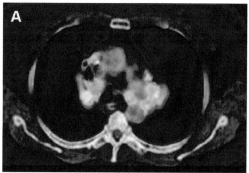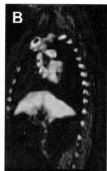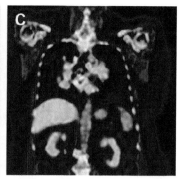

Fig. 3. ^{18}F-FDG PET/CT for CS axial (*A*), sagittal (*B*), and coronal (*C*) chest images, demonstrating extracardiac manifesting as 18F-FDG-avid hilar lymphadenopathy.

CS manifests as patchy or focal on diffuse ^{18}F-FDG uptake, which may or may not have correspondent myocardial perfusion abnormalities. Care should be taken to not misinterpret focal ^{18}F-FDG surrounding implantable cardiac leads as pathologic[39] or isolated lateral ^{18}F-FDG uptake, which may be a nonspecific finding.[8] Quantitative assessment of myocardial inflammation by determination of ^{18}F-FDG standard uptake value (SUV) is an area of active research interest. Initial studies have demonstrated the determination of SUV may improve ^{18}F-FDG PET/CT specificity for the detection of CS without compromising sensitivity.[30,40] Currently, however, there is no specific SUV threshold that can be used to delineate inflamed from normal myocardial tissue.

After assessment of the myocardial perfusion and inflammatory images, extracardiac structures should be evaluated for both areas of sarcoid involvement and for incident findings. With the advent of CT as the transmission source for PET imaging, it has been reported that as many as half of all cardiac studies contain an extracardiac incidental finding worth including in the final report.[41–43] Finally, if available, prior PET/CT CS studies should be compared for any change because this may have implications for subsequent clinical decision making.

CLINICAL RELEVANCE OF THE PET/CT CARDIAC SARCOIDOSIS STUDY

The results of the PET/CT examination have diagnostic, prognostic, and therapeutic ramifications. In regard to diagnosis, PET/CT has the highest diagnostic accuracy among both invasive and noninvasive techniques, with a meta-analysis of 7 studies involving 164 patients with systemic sarcoidosis reporting a sensitivity of 89% and a specificity of 78%.[44] In terms of prognosis, the combination of both a perfusion and ^{18}F-FDG abnormality portends a worse outcome ,with a reported 4-fold increase in the annual rate of malignant arrhythmias and mortality compared with patients with normal images.[45] This finding remains significant even after adjusting for left ventricular ejection fraction and clinical variables. Furthermore, abnormal right ventricular ^{18}F-FDG uptake also demonstrated a significant negative influence on patient outcomes.[45] Using PET/CT to assess therapeutic response is also of great interest. A study of 95 patients demonstrated initiation of immunosuppressive therapy prior to deterioration in cardiac systolic function resulted in excellent clinical outcomes.[46] Additional investigations demonstrated that reduction of ^{18}F-FDG after initiation of therapy, as noted on PET/CT imaging, correlated with improvement in left ventricular ejection fraction as well as a decrease in major associated cardiovascular events.[47,48] Furthermore, Muser and colleagues[49] have demonstrated the utility of PET/CT imaging in assessing the CS patient prior to electrophysiologic anatomic mapping and potential ablation therapy, noting that abnormal electrograms were more likely in areas of a lower degree of inflammation as determined by PET and that a positive PET/CT for CS at baseline or lack of improvement on serial PET/CT imaging portended worse arrhythmia-free survivals in patients undergoing catheter ablation therapy.[50] Standard methodology for determining changes from one PET/CT study to another for the CS patient is lacking. Attempts have been made to implement quantitative techniques in the form of comparing SUV maximum as well as the total volume of myocardium demonstrating abnormal ^{18}F-FDG uptake between serial examinations.[25,47,51] What constitutes a meaningful change in SUV, however, is uncertain, with some investigators proposing that at least a 20% difference should be seen before declaring a difference between studies.[25] Further investigations are required to help clarify what constitutes a therapeutic response or failure.

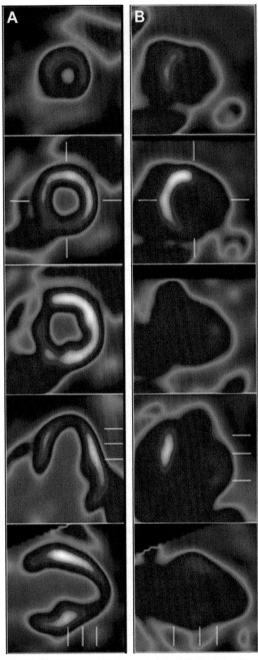

Fig. 4. ^{18}F-FDG and N-13 ammonia PET/CT for CS. A myocardial perfusion defect is present in the septum on N-13 ammonia imaging (*A*) with corresponding ^{18}F-FDG uptake in the same territory (*B*) consistent with active CS.

PET/CT COMPARED WITH ALTERNATIVE IMAGING MODALITIES FOR THE DETECTION OF CARDIAC SARCOIDOSIS

Alternatives to PET/CT imaging for the assessment of CS include single-photon emission CT (SPECT), echocardiography, and MR imaging. In regard to SPECT techniques, both technetium Tc 99m (^{99m}Tc) and thallium-201 (^{201}Tl) may demonstrate perfusion defects due to either scar or arteriole constriction secondary to inflammation. If inflammation is present, myocardial perfusion defects may improve or resolve on vasodilator stress imaging (reverse redistribution) due to dilation of the microvasculature that is constricted by inflamed tissue.[52] One study suggested that the finding of reverse redistribution could predict a positive response to immunosuppressive therapy.[53] ^{18}F-FDG PET/CT has a greater sensitivity for the detection of CS than either SPECT ^{99m}Tc-labeled perfusion tracers or SPECT ^{201}Tl and allows for direct detection of inflamed tissues rendering it the preferred modality for this patient population.

Gallium-67 (^{67}Ga) is another SPECT technique that has demonstrated the capability to detect CS. ^{67}Ga is taken up by activated macrophages in inflamed tissue[54] and correlates with both clinical and histologic evidence of CS.[54–56] Furthermore, the presence of ^{67}Ga has therapeutic implications because it is an indicator of steroid responsiveness.[57] Unfortunately, extracardiac uptake of ^{67}Ga may obscure cardiac uptake and thereby limit test sensitivity to less than 40%.[58] Modest improvements to sensitivity have been demonstrated with the concurrent use of ^{99m}Tc-labeled perfusion tracers to delineate the heart; however, sensitivity reaches only 68% with this technique, which unfortunately also entails higher patient radiation exposure.[58,59]

Echocardiography and MR imaging are among the non-nuclear imaging modalities that have been used to assess CS. Cited echocardiographic characteristics of CS include thinning of the basal interventricular septal and regional wall motion abnormalities with or without aneurysm in territories not consistent with a coronary distribution.[5,6] These findings are often not seen until the late stages of CS, however, and have a very low reported sensitivity of 25%.[60] T1-weighted and T2-weighted cardiac MR imaging sequences can be used to detect myocardial inflammation and scar, with sensitivity and specificity of 75% for CS.[61] MR imaging findings also have prognostic and therapeutic importance, as evident in a study demonstrating a 20-fold increase in mortality in patients with abnormal delayed enhancement[61] whereas others have also noted a correlation between decreased delayed enhancement and a positive response to immunosuppressive therapy.[62,63] A particular benefit of MR imaging compared with PET/CT imaging is that it does

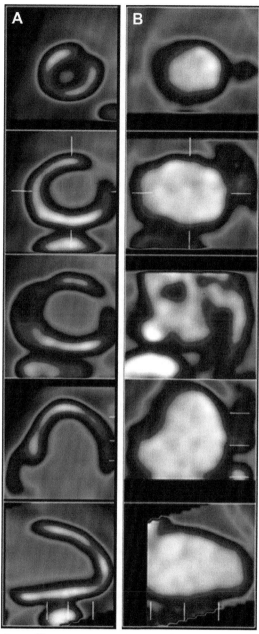

Fig. 5. ^{18}F-FDG and N-13 ammonia PET/CT for CS. A myocardial perfusion defect is present in the apical and anterolateral wall at the mid and base on N-13 ammonia imaging (*A*) without corresponding pathologic ^{18}F-FDG uptake consistent with scar from prior disease (*B*).

not expose patients to ionizing radiation. Limitations of MR imaging, however, include incompatibility with some intracardiac devices, contraindication in severe renal failure, limited accessibility, and difficulty in performing the test for patients who suffer from claustrophobia.

DEVELOPING ADVANCES IN PET IMAGING OF CARDIAC SARCOIDOSIS

Several advances in PET imaging of CS, including the potential use of alternative inflammatory radiotracers in the form of ^{68}Ga-DOTATATE[32,33] as well as the ongoing attempts to quantify inflammatory burden through calculation of SUV,[30,40] have been addressed previously.[30,32,33,40] Additional developing areas of interest include MBF quantification and the coupling of PET with MR imaging to perform hybrid PET/MR imaging of CS.

Recent technological advances in myocardial PET imaging have allowed for more routine quantification of MBF (mL/g/min) and myocardial flow reserve (MBF at stress/MBF at rest). In patients with known or suspected coronary artery disease, MBF has proved both reproducible and accurate while also adding incremental diagnostic and prognostic value.[64,65] Studying a small CS population of 32 patients, Kruse and colleagues[66] demonstrated that MFR was decreased in myocardial segments afflicted by active CS disease and that global MFR was decreased in patients who did not responded to immunosuppressive therapy compared with those who did. Further investigations are needed to validate these findings and to assess the potential role of MBF and MFR in the CS population.

Advancements in semiconductor technology have allowed for the creation of hybrid PET/MR imaging.[67] In the CS population, the hope is that the coregistration of the metabolic imaging capabilities of PET with the morphologic, functional, and tissue imaging of MR imaging may improve diagnostic accuracy and potentially provide further prognostic and therapeutic insights.[68] Initial feasibility studies using the hybrid PET/MR imaging technique have been promising (see **Fig. 5**).[30] Potential challenges for the implementation of hybrid PET/MR imaging are both technical, including the need to refine MR imaging attenuation methods[69] and optimizing acquisition protocols, and practical, including demonstrating that such a hybrid technique provides incremental benefits to the care of the CS patient beyond traditional imaging techniques.

SUMMARY

Accurate diagnosis of CS is critical for diagnostic, therapeutic, and prognostic purposes. Cardiac PET/CT has emerged as the leading modality by which to detect CS. Effective performance of PET/CT for CS entails knowledge of appropriate indications, patient preparation, study performance, and interpretation and its ultimate bearing on clinical care. Further advances in the technique, including alternative metabolic radiotracers, quantification of MBF, and inflammation and potential hybridization are actively being explored and could further enhance the capabilities of PET imaging.

REFERENCES

1. Dumas O, Abramovitz L, Wiley AS, et al. Epidemiology of sarcoidosis in a prospective cohort study of U.S. women. Ann Am Thorac Soc 2016;13(1):67–71.

2. Erdal BS, Clymer BD, Yildiz VO, et al. Unexpectedly high prevalence of sarcoidosis in a representative U.S. Metropolitan population. Respir Med 2012; 106(6):893–9.

3. Statement on sarcoidosis. Joint Statement of the American Thoracic Society (ATS), the European Respiratory Society (ERS) and the World Association of Sarcoidosis and Other Granulomatous Disorders (WASOG) adopted by the ATS Board of Directors and by the ERS Executive Committee, February 1999. Am J Respir Crit Care Med 1999; 160(2):736–55.

4. Silverman KJ, Hutchins GM, Bulkley BH. Cardiac sarcoid: a clinicopathologic study of 84 unselected patients with systemic sarcoidosis. Circulation 1978;58(6):1204–11.

5. Perry A, Vuitch F. Causes of death in patients with sarcoidosis. A morphologic study of 38 autopsies with clinicopathologic correlations. Arch Pathol Lab Med 1995;119(2):167–72.

6. Doughan AR, Williams BR. Cardiac sarcoidosis. Heart 2006;92(2):282–8.

7. Nensa F, Poeppel TD, Krings P, et al. Multiparametric assessment of myocarditis using simultaneous positron emission tomography/magnetic resonance imaging. Eur Heart J 2014;35(32):2173.

8. Chareonthaitawee P, Beanlands RS, Chen W, et al. Joint SNMMI-ASNC expert consensus document on the role of (18)F-FDG PET/CT in cardiac sarcoid detection and therapy monitoring. J Nucl Med 2017;58(8):1341–53.

9. Yoshinaga TFAK. New guidelines for diagnosis of cardiac sarcoidosis in Japan. Annals of Nuclear Cardiology 2017.

10. Birnie DH, Sauer WH, Bogun F, et al. HRS expert consensus statement on the diagnosis and management of arrhythmias associated with cardiac sarcoidosis. Heart Rhythm 2014;11(7):1305–23.

11. Bois JP, Chareonthaitawee P. Continuing evolution in preparation protocols for 18FDG PET assessment of inflammatory or malignant myocardial disease. J Nucl Cardiol 2017;24(3):989–92.

12. Camici P, Ferrannini E, Opie LH. Myocardial metabolism in ischemic heart disease: basic principles and application to imaging by positron emission tomography. Prog Cardiovasc Dis 1989;32(3):217–38.

13. Taegtmeyer H, Overturf ML. Effects of moderate hypertension on cardiac function and metabolism in the rabbit. Hypertension 1988;11(5):416–26.

14. Maurer AH, Burshteyn M, Adler LP, et al. How to differentiate benign versus malignant cardiac and paracardiac 18F FDG uptake at oncollogic PET/CT. Radiographics 2011;31:1287–305.

15. Taegtmeyer H. Tracing cardiac metabolism in vivo: one substrate at a time. J Nucl Med 2010;51(Suppl 1):80S–7S.

16. Manabe O, Yoshinaga K, Ohira H, et al. The effects of 18-h fasting with low-carbohydrate diet preparation on suppressed physiological myocardial (18)F-fluorodeoxyglucose (FDG) uptake and possible minimal effects of unfractionated heparin use in patients with suspected cardiac involvement sarcoidosis. J Nucl Cardiol 2016;23(2):244–52.

17. Masuda A, Naya M, Manabe O, et al. Administration of unfractionated heparin with prolonged fasting could reduce physiological 18F-fluorodeoxyglucose uptake in the heart. Acta Radiol 2016;57(6):661–8.

18. Morooka M, Moroi M, Uno K, et al. Long fasting is effective in inhibiting physiological myocardial 18F-FDG uptake and for evaluating active lesions of cardiac sarcoidosis. EJNMMI Res 2014;4(1):1.

19. Langah R, Spicer K, Gebregziabher M, et al. Effectiveness of prolonged fasting 18f-FDG PET-CT in the detection of cardiac sarcoidosis. J Nucl Cardiol 2009;16(5):801–10.

20. Kyrtatos PG, Constandinou N, Loizides S, et al. Improved patient education facilitates adherence to preoperative fasting guidelines. J Perioper Pract 2014;24(10):228–31.

21. Nadella V, GM, Brown J, et al. Evaluation of adherence to recommended fasting guidelines in pediatric surgery in a teaching hospital in the UKL 19AP3-3. Eur J Anaesthesiol 2013;30:162–3.

22. Harisankar CN, Mittal BR, Agrawal KL. Utility of high fat and low carbohydrate diet in suppressing myocardial FDG uptake. J Nucl Cardiol 2011;18(5):926–36.

23. Wisneski JA, Gertz EW, Neese RA, et al. Myocardial metabolism of free fatty acids. Studies with 14C-labeled substrates in humans. J Clin Invest 1987; 79(2):359–66.

24. Gormsen LC, Christensen NL, Bendstrup E, et al. Complete somatostatin-induced insulin suppression combined with heparin loading does not significantly suppress myocardial 18F-FDG uptake in patients with suspected cardiac sarcoidosis. J Nucl Cardiol 2013;20(6):1108–15.

25. Waller AH, Blankstein R. Quantifying myocardial inflammation using F18-fluorodeoxyglucose positron emission tomography in cardiac sarcoidosis. J Nucl Cardiol 2014;21(5):940–3.

26. Osborne MT, Hulten EA, Murthy VL, et al. Patient preparation for cardiac fluorine-18 fluorodeoxyglucose positron emission tomography imaging of inflammation. J Nucl Cardiol 2017;24(1):86–99.

27. Bois JP, Chareonthaitawee P. Patient page-sarcoidosis imaging. J Nucl Cardiol 2017. [Epub ahead of print].

28. Bois JP, Chareonthaitawee P. Optimizing radionuclide imaging in the assessment of cardiac sarcoidosis. J Nucl Cardiol 2016;23(2):253–5.

29. Ishida Y, Yoshinaga K, Miyagawa M, et al. Recommendations for (18)F-fluorodeoxyglucose positron emission tomography imaging for cardiac sarcoidosis: Japanese Society of Nuclear Cardiology recommendations. Ann Nucl Med 2014;28(4):393–403.

30. Nensa F, Tezgah E, Schweins K, et al. Evaluation of a low-carbohydrate diet-based preparation protocol without fasting for cardiac PET/MR imaging. J Nucl Cardiol 2017;24(3):980–8.

31. Mojtahedi A, Thamake S, Tworowska I, et al. The value of (68)Ga-DOTATATE PET/CT in diagnosis and management of neuroendocrine tumors compared to current FDA approved imaging modalities: a review of literature. Am J Nucl Med Mol Imaging 2014;4(5):426–34.

32. Gormsen LC, Haraldsen A, Kramer S, et al. A dual tracer (68)Ga-DOTANOC PET/CT and (18)F-FDG PET/CT pilot study for detection of cardiac sarcoidosis. EJNMMI Res 2016;6(1):52.

33. Lapa C, Reiter T, Kircher M, et al. Somatostatin receptor based PET/CT in patients with the suspicion of cardiac sarcoidosis: an initial comparison to cardiac MRI. Oncotarget 2016;7(47):77807–14.

34. Dilsizian V, Bacharach SL, Beanlands RS, et al. ASNC imaging guidelines/SNMMI procedure standard for positron emission tomography (PET) nuclear cardiology procedures. J Nucl Cardiol 2016; 23(5):1187–226.

35. Delso G, Furst S, Jakoby B, et al. Performance measurements of the Siemens mMR integrated whole-body PET/MR scanner. J Nucl Med 2011;52(12): 1914–22.

36. Gould KL, Pan T, Loghin C, et al. Frequent diagnostic errors in cardiac PET/CT due to misregistration of CT attenuation and emission PET images: a definitive analysis of causes, consequences, and corrections. J Nucl Med 2007;48(7):1112–21.

37. Blankstein R, Waller AH. Evaluation of known or suspected cardiac sarcoidosis. Circ Cardiovasc Imaging 2016;9(3):e000867.

38. Okumura W, Iwasaki T, Toyama T, et al. Usefulness of fasting 18F-FDG PET in identification of cardiac sarcoidosis. J Nucl Med 2004;45(12):1989–98.

39. DiFilippo FP, Brunken RC. Do implanted pacemaker leads and ICD leads cause metal-related artifact in cardiac PET/CT? J Nucl Med 2005;46(3):436–43.

40. Tahara N, Tahara A, Nitta Y, et al. Heterogenous myocardial FDG uptake and the disease activity in cardiac sarcoidosis. JACC Cardiovasc Imaging 2010;3(12):1219–28.

41. Douglas PS, Cerqueria M, Rubin GD, et al. Extracardiac findings: what is a cardiologist to do? JACC Cardiovasc Imaging 2008;1(5):682–7.

42. Husmann L, Tatsugami F, Buechel RR, et al. Incidental detection of a pulmonary adenocarcinoma on low-dose computed tomography used for attenuation correction in myocardial perfusion imaging with SPECT. Clin Nucl Med 2010;35(9):751–2.

43. Shawgi M, Arumugam P. Looking outside the "cardiac" box: incidental detection of a metastatic lung tumor on cardiac position emission tomography/computed tomography. World J Nucl Med 2014; 13(3):197–200.

44. Youssef G, Leung E, Mylonas I, et al. The use of 18F-FDG PET in the diagnosis of cardiac sarcoidosis: a systematic review and metaanalysis including the Ontario experience. J Nucl Med 2012;53(2):241–8.

45. Blankstein R, Osborne M, Naya M, et al. Cardiac positron emission tomography enhances prognostic assessments of patients with suspected cardiac sarcoidosis. J Am Coll Cardiol 2014;63(4):329–36.

46. Yazaki Y, Isobe M, Hiroe M, et al. Prognostic determinants of long-term survival in Japanese patients with cardiac sarcoidosis treated with prednisone. Am J Cardiol 2001;88(9):1006–10.

47. Osborne MT, Hulten EA, Singh A, et al. Reduction in 18F-fluorodeoxyglucose uptake in serial cardiac positrom emission tomography is associated with improved left ventricualr ejection fraction in patients with cardiac sarcoidosis. J Nucl Cardiol 2014; 2014(21):166–74.

48. Muser D, Santangeli P, Castro SA, et al. Prognostic role of serial quantitative evaluation of (18)F-fluorodeoxyglucose uptake by PET/CT in patients with cardiac sarcoidosis presenting with ventricular tachycardia. Eur J Nucl Med Mol Imaging 2018; 45(8):1394–404.

49. Muser D, Santangeli P, Liang J, et al. Characterization of the electroanatomic substrate in cardiac sarcoidosis, vol. 4, 2017.

50. Muser D, Santangeli P, Pathak RK, et al. Long-term outcomes of catheter ablation of ventricular tachycardia in patients with cardiac sarcoidosis. Circ Arrhythm Electrophysiol 2016;9(8) [pii:e004333].

51. Ahmadian A, Pawar S, Govender P, et al. The response of FDG uptake to immunosuppressive treatment on FDG PET/CT imaging for cardiac sarcoidosis. J Nucl Cardiol 2017;24(2):413–24.

52. Tawarahara K, Kurata C, Okayama K, et al. Thallium-201 and gallium 67 single photon emission computed tomographic imaging in cardiac sarcoidosis. Am Heart J 1992;124(5):1383–4.

53. Matsui Y, Iwai K, Tachibana T, et al. Clinicopatholog-ical study of fatal myocardial sarcoidosis. Ann N Y Acad Sci 1976;278:455–69.

54. Maná J, Kroonenburgh M. Clinical usefulness of nu-clear imaging techniques in sarcoidosis, vol. 32, 2005.

55. Hirose Y, Ishida Y, Hayashida K, et al. Myocardial involvement in patients with sarcoidosis. An analysis of 75 patients. Clin Nucl Med 1994;19(6):522–6.

56. Okamoto H, Mizuno K, Ohtoshi E. Cutaneous sarcoidosis with cardiac involvement. Eur J Derma-tol 1999;9(6):466–9.

57. Okayama K, Kurata C, Tawarahara K, et al. Diag-nostic and prognostic value of myocardial scintig-raphy with thallium-201 and gallium-67 in cardiac sarcoidosis. Chest 1995;107(2):330–4.

58. Nakazawa A, Ikeda K, Ito Y, et al. Usefulness of dual 67Ga and 99mTc-sestamibi single-photon-emission CT scanning in the diagnosis of cardiac sarcoidosis. Chest 2004;126(4):1372–6.

59. Mana J, Gamez C. Molecular imaging in sarcoid-osis. Curr Opin Pulm Med 2011;17(5):325–31.

60. Cooper LT, Baughman KL, Feldman AM, et al. The role of endomyocardial biopsy in the management of cardiovascular disease: a scientific statement from the American Heart Association, the American College of Cardiology, and the European Society of Cardiology. Endorsed by the Heart Failure Society of America and the Heart Failure Association of the European Society of Cardiology. J Am Coll Cardiol 2007;50(19):1914–31.

61. Ohira H, Tsujino I, Ishimaru S, et al. Myocardial im-aging with 18F-fluoro-2-deoxyglucose positron emission tomography and magnetic resonance imaging in sarcoidosis. Eur J Nucl Med Mol Imaging 2008;35(5):933–41.

62. Sekiguchi M, Yazaki Y, Isobe M, et al. Cardiac sarcoidosis: diagnostic, prognostic, and therapeutic considerations. Cardiovasc Drugs Ther 1996;10(5): 495–510.

63. Vignaux O, Dhote R, Duboc D, et al. Clinical signifi-cance of myocardial magnetic resonance abnormal-ities in patients with sarcoidosis: a 1-year follow-up study. Chest 2002;122(6):1895–901.

64. Herzog BA, Husmann L, Valenta I, et al. Long-term prognostic value of 13N-ammonia myocardial perfu-sion positron emission tomography added value of coronary flow reserve. J Am Coll Cardiol 2009; 54(2):150–6.

65. Chareonthaitawee P, Christenson SD, Anderson JL, et al. Reproducibility of measurements of regional myocardial blood flow in a model of coronary artery disease: comparison of H2150 and 13NH3 PET techniques. J Nucl Med 2006;47(7):1193–201.

66. Kruse MJ, Kovell L, Kasper EK, et al. Myocardial blood flow and inflammatory cardiac sarcoidosis. JACC Cardiovasc Imaging 2017;10(2):157–67.

67. LaForest R, Woodard PK, Gropler RJ. Cardiovascu-lar PET/MRI: challenges and opportunities. Cardiol Clin 2016;34(1):25–35.

68. White JA, Rajchl M, Butler J, et al. Active cardiac sarcoidosis: first clinical experience of simultaneous positron emission tomography–magnetic resonance imaging for the diagnosis of cardiac disease. Circu-lation 2013;127(22):e639–41.

69. Coombs BD, Szumowski J, Coshow W. Two-point Dixon technique for water-fat signal decomposition with B0 inhomogeneity correction. Magn Reson Med 1997;38(6):884–9.

PET/MR Imaging in Cardiovascular Imaging

Christoph Rischpler, MD[a],*, Pamela K. Woodard, MD[b]

KEYWORDS

- PET/MR imaging • Cardiovascular • Molecular imaging • FDG

KEY POINTS

- Hybrid PET/MR imaging is a complex yet highly valuable tool in cardiovascular imaging.
- Hybrid PET/MR imaging's value has been established for myocardial viability imaging and for imaging inflammatory processes in the heart, and it serves as an important research tool for cross-validation of 2 imaging modalities (eg, in myocardial perfusion imaging).
- Further studies are warranted in the field of atherosclerotic plaque imaging, where only small studies and case reports are available.

INTRODUCTION

Before PET/computed tomography (CT) appeared on the market, nuclear cardiology was restricted to single-photon emission computed tomography (SPECT) imaging. Although the success of PET/CT mainly attributed its broad application in oncology, as a consequence, PET/CT scanners were also available for application in other fields, including nuclear cardiology. In analogy to this, more and more PET/MR imaging scanners have now been installed in imaging centers and researchers with a focus on cardiovascular imaging benefit from this trend. Today, more than 70 PET/MR imaging scanners, most of them simultaneous PET/MR imaging scanners (Siemens Biograph mMR or GE SIGNA), have been installed worldwide, and users of this technology expect an increase in its utilization in cardiovascular imaging.

The most promising applications include viability imaging of hypoperfused or ischemically compromised myocardium and imaging of myocardial inflammation. In addition, PET/MR imaging has been identified as a good tool for cross-validation of parameters accessible both by PET and MR imaging such as myocardial perfusion.

Last but not the least, the utilization of PET/MR imaging in conjunction with novel radiotracers has been suggested for imaging a variety of molecular targets such as those expressed in angiogenesis or subgroups of inflammatory cells in atherosclerotic plaque and the myocardium. Disadvantages to PET/MR imaging include a more complex workflow and the high cost of the scanner and associated maintenance.

In this review, the authors give an overview of PET/MR imaging technical updates and discuss the most promising applications in the cardiovascular field.

Technical Aspects of PET/MR imaging

The high electromagnetic field and rapidly switching gradient coils and radiofrequency signals of MR imaging are known to interfere with photomultiplier tubes and electronics in "traditional" PET scanners. Moreover, PET detectors may degrade MR image quality by introducing electromagnetic interference and inhomogeneities. Thus, the development of an integrated PET/MR imaging scanner was a time-consuming and costly process. One early approach was the connection of a PET/CT scanner to a stand-alone MR imaging

[a] Department of Nuclear Medicine, University Hospital Essen, University of Duisburg-Essen, Essen, Germany;
[b] Mallinckrodt Institute of Radiology, Washington University School of Medicine, St Louis, MO, USA
* Corresponding author.
E-mail address: Christoph.Rischpler@uk-essen.de

PET Clin 14 (2019) 233–244
https://doi.org/10.1016/j.cpet.2018.12.005
1556-8598/19/© 2018 Elsevier Inc. All rights reserved.

via a movable table system. This was first implemented by Philips as the Ingenuity TF PET/MR system.[1] A second truly integrated approach that placed the PET system directly into the MR imaging scanner (Siemens Biograph mMR,[2] GE SIGNA PET/MR[3]) required the construction of novel detectors. Siemens first used avalanche photodiodes (ie, photodetectors made of lutetium oxyorthosilicate crystal), insensitive to magnetic fields,[4] while GE then followed with silicon photomultiplier technology–based PET detectors, which allow time-of-flight PET imaging with a temporal resolution of less than 400 picoseconds.[5] A major issue of the integration of PET into an MR imaging tube was the generation of an attenuation correction (AC) map to correct PET images. This step is mandatory for quantitative PET imaging and therefore of utmost importance in cardiovascular PET.

Estimation of tissue attenuation in PET/MR imaging

In traditional stand-alone PET systems, attenuation of surrounding tissues was estimated by rotating rod sources (eg, Germanium-68). In integrated PET/CT systems, attenuation is estimated using a CT data μ-map. Because Hounsfield units (HU) directly correlate with tissue density, AC μ-maps may be generated quickly and accurately. Because MR imaging data do not necessarily correlate with tissue density, novel approaches to generate AC maps for 511 keV photons had to be developed.

Usually, AC μ-maps are generated from MR data sets using templates, segmentation approaches, or atlases. Some approaches also use non-AC PET datasets to estimate certain parts of the AC map. In the segmentation approach, the body is segmented into different tissue classes to which certain fixed attenuation coefficients for 511 keV photons are assigned.[6] In the Siemens Biograph, the segmentation is performed based on water and fat images from a DIXON VIBE sequence, which in turn allows the definition of air, lung, fat, and soft tissue.[7,8] In severely ill patients, this method may not be achievable because this sequence requires an 18-second breath-hold for each bed position. There are alternative approaches with a T1-weighted turbo spin echo sequence with shorter acquisition times; however, fat and soft tissue differences (0.086 cm^{-1} vs 0.096 cm^{-1}) with regard to attenuation are ignored.[9] It is now possible to also model bone by the application of an atlas as recently implemented in the Siemens mMR system.[10] In the Philips Ingenuity TF T1w-GE MR, images are used for the segmentation of 3 different tissue classes (air, lung, and soft tissue). In the GE Signa PET/MR imaging,

similar to the Siemens approach, the body is segmented into air, lung, fat, and soft tissue using a multistation, whole-body, 3-dimensional, dual-echo, radiofrequency-spoiled gradient recalled echo sequence (LAVA-Flex).[11] It becomes obvious that the constraint to a limited number of tissue classes may cause deviations in the assessment of radiotracer uptake. For instance, for thoracic tumors, radiotracer uptake on PET/MR in comparison to PET/CT may vary in the order of 5% to 23%.[8,9,12] Yet, in cardiovascular applications only minor variations between PET/CT and PET/MR imaging have been reported.[13] A major limitation of these techniques is that the MR field-of-view is often too small to "see" the whole body (particularly parts of the shoulders and arms), resulting in an underestimation of attenuation in this area.[14] To recover these parts of the body in the AC μ-map, the so-called maximum likelihood estimation of activity and attenuation (MLAA) approach using (non-AC) emission PET data are used.[15] MLAA works well with fludeoxyglucose (FDG), because virtually any tissue (also skin and fat) has at least some degree of tracer retention. There are alternative ways to estimate attenuation of surrounding tissues but, because they are not used in current clinically available PET/MR imaging systems, they are not discussed here.[16]

Another very promising update of the Siemens mMR that has recently been introduced is CAIPIRINHA (controlled aliasing in parallel imaging results in higher acceleration), an accelerated Dixon 3D-VIBE sequence, which allows MR imaging with higher resolution at scan-times identical to the VIBE DIXON (19 seconds per bed position).[17] This sequence may be used not only for AC but also for diagnostic purposes, which may allow the elimination of other diagnostic sequences with longer acquisition times. Thus CAIPIRINHA could result in a shorter overall scan-time, increased patient-throughput, and improved cost efficiency, all major limitations of PET/MR imaging in comparison to PET/CT.

Interference by contrast agents and cardiac devices

Cardiac devices (such as sternal wires, pacemakers, defibrillators etc.) may lead to beam-hardening artifacts in CT, which are subsequently transcribed into the AC μ-map and AC-PET data. In these cases, an overestimation of radiotracer uptake is regularly noticed. Hence, clinicians should always examine non-AC PET data, particularly in the case of suspected infection of lead wires (pacemaker, implantable cardiac defibrillator) or prosthetic valves in order to avoid false-positive readings.[18] Conversely, when MR imaging is used for AC, cardiac devices composed of non-ferromagnetic metallic materials usually cause signal voids that exceed the size of the respective device. This in turn causes an underestimation of the attenuation and leads to an underestimation of radiotracer accumulation. A major limitation in cardiovascular PET/MR imaging is that many patients cannot be scanned because they have implanted devices that are not compatible with 3T field strengths. Besides heating of the device, malfunction may occur and therefore every implanted device has to be checked with caution for its compatibility with 3T MR imaging. Many novel cardiac devices have entered the market (to include heart valves, event-recorders, and atrial appendage closure devices), and data on the compatibility of these devices with 3T MR imaging must be thoroughly evaluated before any patient imaging. Often there is limited data available regarding if and to what degree these devices cause artifacts on MR imaging, which could subsequently be translated into AC-corrected PET data. In a recent study, ^{18}F FDG and N-13 ammonia PET/MR imaging scans of 20 patients were analyzed with respect to attenuation artifacts. In patients with sternal wires or metallic implants, artifacts were found in 20% and 30% of the cases, respectively, and the maximum relative difference in the SUV_{mean} ranged from 11% to 196% in ^{18}F FDG or N-13 ammonia AC PET data when correction for these artifacts was performed.[19]

Another fact that has to be considered is that MR contrast agents reduce T_1 values. This T_1 value reduction in turn affects the Dixon VIBE sequence and may cause commonly observed AC μ-map errors[20,21]; thus gadolinium-based MR contrast materials should be administered only after the acquisition of MR AC sequences.

Cardiovascular Applications of Hybrid PET/MR Imaging

Myocardial perfusion imaging

Myocardial perfusion imaging (MPI) using SPECT or PET with its high sensitivity and specificity[22] is still the most often conducted study in nuclear cardiology. It has a high impact on patient management as the following clinically important questions may be answered: primary diagnosis of coronary artery disease, hemodynamic significance of known coronary stenosis, therapy control, extent of ischemia and therapy guidance, risk stratification before noncardiac surgery, or prognostic stratification.[23–26] PET is known to be superior to SPECT because of an intrinsically superior image quality (particularly in obese patients) and the possibility of myocardial blood flow (MBF)

quantification.[27] In the United States, N-13 ammonia and Rubidium-82 are approved by the Food and Drug Administration (FDA) and consequently are the most often applied radiotracers for assessment of myocardial perfusion. O-15 water is another perfusion tracer that has been studied extensively and which is thought to be superior because of its free diffusion and thus "perfect" first pass extraction. However, O-15 water is currently not FDA approved and not reimbursed by insurance companies. Moreover, the Rubidium-82 generator is difficult to use in the MR imaging setting. F-18 flurpiridaz is a very promising perfusion tracer because of its high first-pass extraction of 94%,[28] which has been validated in a first phase II clinical trial.[29] The advantages of F-18 flurpiridaz, in comparison to other radiotracers for cardiac perfusion imaging, are that it has a low positron energy (E_{max} = 634 keV) and does not need either a cost-intensive and MR imaging–noncompatible Rb-82 generator or an onsite cyclotron because of its longer half-life ($T_{1/2}$ = 110 min) in comparison to other myocardial perfusion PET tracers (O-15 water: $T_{1/2}$ = 122 seconds, N-13 ammonia: $T_{1/2}$: 10 minutes). Moreover, an F-18 flurpiridaz preclinical study suggests that MBF calculation remains possible even in the case of radiotracer injection outside of the scanner because simplified quantification models may be feasible.[30,31] This would allow for stress MPI using exercise with the scanning schedule optimized to increase patient throughput because a short static scan, rather than list mode acquisition, would be sufficient.

Over the past decade MR imaging MPI has also been successfully established. One of the biggest advantages of MR imaging MPI is the high spatial resolution potentially capable of unmasking small subendocardial areas of ischemia. The proof-of-principle that first-pass MR imaging with gadolinium-based contrast agents is feasible to detect flow-limiting coronary artery disease was demonstrated in the early 1990s.[32] Its worth in coronary artery disease has since then be confirmed in many studies.[33,34] In the vast majority of these studies, however, only visual analysis was performed, a barrier to the detection of balanced ischemia in advanced coronary artery disease (similar as in SPECT MPI).[35,36] Different approaches in quantifying myocardial blood flow using MR imaging have been undertaken. The upslope ratio as a determination of coronary flow reserve is one of the simplest.[37] However, it has been demonstrated that this method underestimates coronary flow reserve when using N-13 ammonia as a well-established reference method.[38] The central volume principle of quantifying myocardial blood flow[39] is a more complex method that has been used to compare PET and MR imaging MPI in a group of 41 patients.[40] Although good agreement with coronary flow reserve was observed, absolute MBF values showed a high variance using this technique. Recently another work on direct comparison of PET and MR imaging MPI has been published.[41] In this publication using slice average and myocardial segment analysis, a good correlation was found in a group of 29 patients. However, as MR imaging overestimated resting perfusion regardless of the used MR imaging deconvolution method, the coronary flow was low compared with N-13 ammonia PET MPI. In this study it was also demonstrated in one patient with hypertrophic cardiomyopathy that MR imaging, because of its higher spatial resolution in comparison to PET, is capable of differentiating between subepicardial and subendocardial blood flow. Many of the problems of flow quantification with MR imaging lie in the fact that gadolinium-based contrast agents suffer from a low "extraction fraction," which is not solely flow dependent, and that these contrast agents are not accumulated within the cell but distribute in the extracellular volume. Also, MR imaging MPI in clinical routine only images a certain number of slices of the left ventricle (usually 3 short axis) as opposed to PET or SPECT MPI that covers the whole left ventricle. Even though there are approaches to imaging myocardial perfusion of the whole left ventricle using MR imaging,[42] this is not implemented routinely in

clinical practice. Because the extent of myocardial ischemia of the whole left ventricle is key for therapeutic guidance,[25] this is a drawback of MR imaging MPI performed alone.

Hybrid PET/MR imaging, however, allows detection of subendocardial regions of ischemia with MR imaging, whereas PET MPI is the reference standard for absolute perfusion and covers the whole left ventricle. Thus, PET/MR imaging has potential as an ideal tool for cross-validation of novel myocardial perfusion approaches, including novel MR imaging sequences, quantification methods, contrast agents, and radiotracers, with PET MPI as the reference standard. **Fig. 1** depicts a representative workflow for simultaneous PET/MR imaging perfusion imaging both under pharmacologic stress conditions and at rest.

MR angiography and atherosclerotic plaque imaging

The biggest advantage of MR angiography in comparison to CT angiography is that no ionizing radiation is needed.[43,44] In addition, MR vessel wall imaging may provide deeper insights into plaque morphology to include assessment of angiogenesis, hemorrhage, thickness of fibrous cap, or size of the lipid core.[45,46] Of note, several radiotracers have been applied in the performance of molecular imaging of atherosclerotic plaque. [18]F FDG is the most often used radiotracer for this purpose and it has been demonstrated that

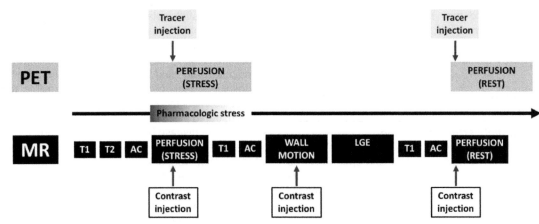

Fig. 1. Representative workflow for simultaneous PET/MR imaging perfusion imaging. *Tracer injection:* slow (preferably pump-driven) tracer injection (eg, O-15 water, Rb-82 or N-13 NH3). Example: N-13 NH3: ≈250 MBq for each study (stress and rest), injection over 30 seconds. *Contrast injection:* in total 0.2 mmol/kgBW ($\frac{1}{4}$ for stress perfusion, $\frac{1}{2}$ for before LGE, $\frac{1}{4}$ for rest perfusion). *Pharmacologic stress:* adenosine (140 µg/kgBW/min over 6 minutes, tracer injection after 3 minutes) or regadenoson (400 µg over 10 s, tracer injection about 30–40 s later), for contraindications cf. guidelines. *PET acquisition:* list mode, gating (ECG and/or respiratory), in the case of N-13 NH3: more than 15 to 20 minutes for each study (stress and rest). *MR acquisition:* gating (ECG and/or respiratory), multiple AC-maps to account for possible patient motion, LGE: 10 to 20 minutes after contrast injection. *Total scan time:* patient inside the scanner for ≈50 to 60 minutes.

its uptake closely correlates with macrophage infiltration, a surrogate marker of plaque vulnerability.[47,48] In a proof-of-principle study, a small number of patients with peripheral artery disease were successfully imaged using hybrid ^{18}F FDG-PET/MR imaging.[49]

More recently, ^{18}F-fluoride (^{18}F-NaF), a radiotracer approved for human use for bone imaging, has been applied to the imaging of atherosclerosis. In a study with 80 patients, 93% of subjects with myocardial infarction demonstrated highest ^{18}F-NaF uptake in the culprit lesion, whereas coronary ^{18}F FDG uptake was often masked by ^{18}F FDG uptake in adjacent myocardium.[50] In 45% of subjects with stable angina, plaques with ^{18}F-NaF uptake were found to also demonstrate high-risk features on intravascular ultrasound. There are many alternative radiotracers with promising targets for plaque vulnerability, such as the integrin

$\alpha_V\beta_3$,[51,52] the alpha-7 nicotine acetylcholine receptor,[53] or the chemokine receptor 4 (CXCR4).[54] In particular, CXCR4 seems to be highly promising as 2 studies have shown a correlation between CXCR4 expression and cardiovascular risk factors.[55,56] It has also been shown that CXCR4 expression is upregulated in culprit coronary artery lesions.[57] In a preclinical study with a rabbit model of atherosclerotic lesions in the aorta and one carotid, PET/MR imaging with Ga-68 pentixafor (a radiotracer targeting CXCR4) was shown to be feasible.[54] Ga-68 pentixafor has been translated into the clinical research setting, imaging patients with severe stenosis of a carotid artery before they underwent endarterectomy (**Fig. 2**). Other chemokine receptors, including CCR5 and CCR2,[58–60] the natriuretic peptide receptor NPR-C,[61–63] and hypoxic macrophages[64,65] have also been identified as potential targets in PET imaging of atherosclerosis.

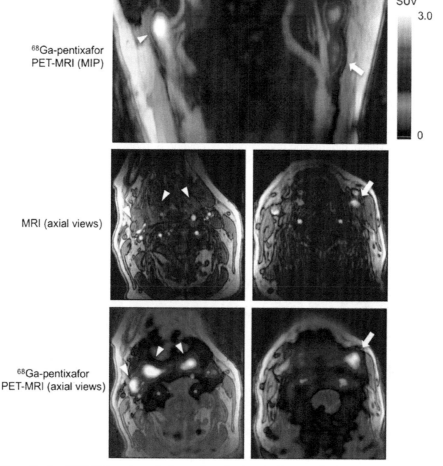

Fig. 2. Ga-68 pentixafor PET/MR imaging of atherosclerotic plaques. Intense CXCR4 expression in an atherosclerotic plaque of a human carotid possibly indicating high vulnerability (*white arrow*). Also note intense CXCR4 expression in lymphoid tissues (adjacent lymph node and tonsils, *white arrowheads*). (*From* Hyafil F, Pelisek J, Laitinen I, et al. Imaging the cytokine receptor CXCR4 in atherosclerotic plaques with the radiotracer 68Ga-Pentixafor for PET. J Nucl Med 2017;58(3):504; with permission.)

So far only small proof-of-principle or retrospective studies exist on this topic. However, hybrid PET/MR imaging seems to be highly promising because MR imaging may be used to correct cardiac and respiratory motion, enabling increase of the usually weak signal of highly specific radiotracers in small lesions in coronary atherosclerotic plaque.[57,66]

Myocardial viability imaging

Myocardial viability imaging is used to image chronically hypoperfused yet viable myocardium, which has shifted its metabolism from fatty acids toward glucose utilization even in the fasting state. Normal myocardium uses either glucose or fatty acids. In the fasting state, normal myocardium predominantly uses fatty acids. In the postprandial state, the myocardium switches to glucose utilization. Hypoperfused regions often demonstrate myocardial viability but contractile dysfunction, a state called "hibernation,"[67] and are likely to recover after revascularization.[68] Hibernating myocardium has prognostic implications because its presence is associated with poor cardiovascular outcome[69] and its presence and extent is important in therapeutic guidance.[70–72] [18]F FDG-PET is an often used method for noninvasive myocardial viability imaging. Cardiac MR late gadolinium-enhanced (LGE) imaging has emerged as an alternative approach. In contrast to ^{18}F FDG-PET, which images viable, hibernating myocardial tissue, LGE MR imaging detects scarred, nonviable, myocardium (**Fig. 3**). Even though the approaches are fundamentally different, a good agreement between the 2 techniques has been shown.[73] An advantage of LGE MR imaging is the high in-plane spatial resolution, which allows differentiation between transmural and nontransmural scarring.[74] In addition, small myocardial scars that are known to have prognostic implications can be detected.[75] PET may not be able to detect small areas of infarction due to its limited spatial resolution. Therefore, a superior tissue classification should be feasible with hybrid PET/MR imaging. According to a meta-analysis, both ^{18}F FDG-PET and LGE MR imaging have a high sensitivity in predicting regional wall motion recovery of more than 90% and 80%, respectively, with acceptable specificity of more than 60%.[76]

Analyses of ^{18}F FDG-PET/MR imaging for viability imaging in the literature is still rare with only 3 published studies.[77–79] Agreement between the 2 modalities has been reported to be moderate to substantial. The addition of ^{18}F FDG-PET to LGE MR imaging resulted in a reclassification of 19% of segments in a publication on a very small cohort of patients.[78] Importantly, no follow-up data were available to study the impact of this reclassification on regional wall motion recovery or other outcome parameters. Also of note is that the PET/MR imaging examinations for viability in the 2 other studies were performed early after revascularization in patients with myocardial infarction. In the study by the Technical University of Munich, the aim was to compare LGE MR imaging and ^{18}F FDG-PET in terms of the prognostic impact on regional recovery 6 months after percutaneous coronary intervention.[77] Intermethod agreement with respect to LGE transmurality and reduction in FDG uptake in the affected segments was high (Cohen K = 0.65). [18]F FDG-PET viable and LGE MR imaging viable segments with wall motion

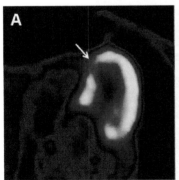 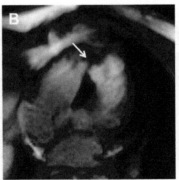 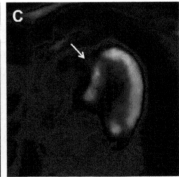

Fig. 3. Colocalization of late gadolinium enhancement (LGE) and reduced FDG-PET activity in an anteroseptal wall myocardial infarction by simultaneous PET/MR acquisition. Cardiac PET /MR imaging in a 65-year-old man with a septal wall myocardial infarction. (*A*) ^{18}F FDG-PET 4-chamber long-axis PET reconstruction shows focal region of decreased radiotracer uptake (*arrow*) that colocalizes to the area of scar shown by (*B*) increased contrast enhancement (*arrow*) on a T1-weighted segmented gradient recalled echo LGE MR image. (*C*) Fused ^{18}F FDG-PET and LGE MR images. (*From* Lau JM, Laforest R, Nensa F, et al. Cardiac applications of PET/MR imaging. Magn Reson Imaging Clin N Am 2017;25(2):325–33; with permission.)

abnormalities were more likely to recover at follow-up at 6 months. Interestingly, some dysfunctional segments with discordant ^{18}F FDG-PET and LGE MR imaging findings were reported. Only 40% of those segments with decreased FDG uptake but only minor LGE findings demonstrated wall motion recovery at follow-up. In another study that was published by the same group, ^{18}F FDG uptake alteration in the ischemically compromised myocardium was compared with LGE MR imaging infarct size and with the area at risk assessed by the endocardial surface area method.[80] The area at risk was shown to be larger in extent in comparison to the infarction area (31% ± 11 vs 10% ± 10). Interestingly, the area at risk was associated with reduced glucose metabolism indicating that revascularized myocardium after myocardial infarction shows a reduction in ^{18}F FDG uptake. The pathophysiologic reason for this finding, namely a metabolic alteration of postischemic myocardium, is unclear and warrants further investigation.

Of note, no study to date has been published with the aim of investigating the prognostic impact of ^{18}F FDG viability PET/MR imaging on left ventricular recovery with imaging before revascularization (eg, in patients with ischemic heart failure) in order to study the additional value of a combined PET/MR imaging approach.

Inflammation imaging of the heart

With MR imaging, multiple processes that suggest or are associated with myocardial inflammation including myocardial edema (T2-weighted imaging) and leaky myocytes or fibrosis (LGE or T1 mapping) can be assessed.[81] Associate processes such as pericardial effusion or wall motion abnormalities may also be present. The use of ^{18}F FDG-PET has recently increased in imaging inflammatory processes in the cardiovascular system.[82] Advantages of ^{18}F FDG-PET are that the extension and grade of the respective inflammatory process may be detected and monitored enabling the differentiation between active and healed inflammatory processes. As described earlier in the section on viability, ^{18}F FDG may also be taken up by viable cardiomyocytes. In order to circumvent this issue, it is important to switch the heart's metabolism away from carbohydrates and toward the consumption of free fatty acids. The most often applied approaches include a high-fat low-carb diet on the day before the scan, prolonged fasting of the patient (eg, >12 hour), and preinjection of heparin before ^{18}F FDG administration.[83,84] In the case of successful preparation, the carbohydrate metabolism of the healthy, noninflamed myocardium is suppressed. FDG uptake in this state indicates pathologic processes, such as inflammation, to include cardiac sarcoidosis or myocarditis. In diabetic patients on certain medications (such as steroids), or in noncompliant subjects, these approaches may fail. As a consequence, the PET community is waiting for and working on radiotracers more specifically targeting inflammatory processes.[85]

[18]F FDG-PET/MR imaging has already been shown to be highly clinically relevant in patients with suspicion of myocarditis. Promising case reports show anecdotal evidence that hybrid ^{18}F FDG-PET/MR imaging can diagnose, grade, and monitor myocarditis.[86–88] In addition, a clinical study of 65 patients with suspected myocarditis imaged by ^{18}F FDG-PET/MR imaging[89] showed a sensitivity of 74% and a specificity of 97% for myocarditis in comparison to a variant of the "Lake Louise Criteria" as reference. An important finding of this study was that patients can have biopsy-proven myocarditis reflected by ^{18}F FDG uptake but without corresponding evidence of myocardial damage on MR imaging, likely identifying myocarditis in an early stage of the disease process (**Fig. 4**). Whether or not combined ^{18}F FDG-PET/MR imaging results in improved and early diagnosis of myocarditis and whether this early detection has an impact on patient outcome still warrants further investigation.[90,91]

Sarcoidosis represents another inflammatory disease process with potential myocardial involvement where ^{18}F FDG-PET/MR imaging may be of importance. Because an increasing number of studies indicate a high value of ^{18}F FDG-PET for the diagnosis, monitoring, and therapy guidance of cardiac sarcoid, this imaging modality has been recommended by an expert consensus.[92] When FDG-PET is accompanied by a perfusion study (eg, N-13 ammonia PET or Tc-99m sestamibi), differentiation between stages of the disease process (early, advanced or healed) is feasible.[93] So far only a few case reports or smaller studies investigating ^{18}F FDG-PET/MR imaging in the case of suspected cardiac sarcoidosis are available.[94–97]

A novel, prognostically relevant marker regarding left ventricular remodeling after myocardial infarction is the postischemic inflammatory response in the heart, which is regulated by different (subsets) of immune cells.[98] The local inflammation of the postischemic heart, which seems to be independent of other established prognostic factors such as infarct size or volume and pressure conditions, may only be assessed by noninvasive imaging.[98–100] Initially, this phenomenon was shown in a rodent model of

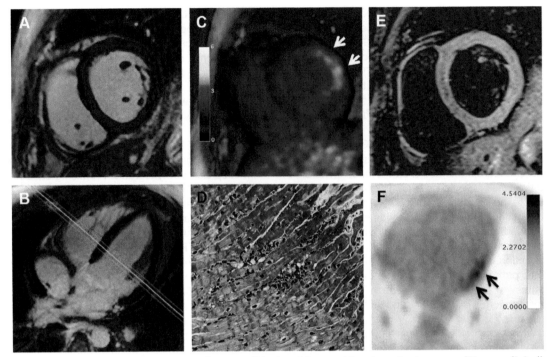

Fig. 4. FDG-PET/MR imaging in suspected myocarditis. In a 30-year-old male patient, myocarditis was clinically suspected due to symptoms such as chest pain, dyspnea, and mild electrocardiogram abnormalities. LGE images (*A, B*) did not demonstrate any pathologies. T2-weighted MR imaging (*E*) demonstrated slight myocardial edema. PET showed clearly an increased FDG uptake of the lateral wall highly suspicious for active inflammation (*C, F*) (*arrows* indicate increased FDG uptake). Endomyocardial biopsy proved the diagnosis of borderline myocarditis (*D*). (*From* Nensa F, Kloth J, Tezgah E, et al. Feasibility of FDG-PET in myocarditis: comparison to CMR using integrated PET/MRI. J Nucl Cardiol 2018;25:785; with permission.)

myocardial infarction using preclinical FDG-PET/MR imaging.[101] However, this imaging technique has subsequently been translated into humans,[102] demonstrating that ^{18}F FDG uptake in the postischemic heart is a prognostic marker for the deterioration of left ventricular pump function after myocardial infarction, independent of infarct size.[103]

This study demonstrates that ^{18}F FDG-PET/MR imaging can serve as a tool to assess the individual risk of ventricular remodeling in patients after myocardial infarction, with the potential to be used in assessment of interventions designed to slow or halt the remodeling process.

SUMMARY

For a long period of time the construction of an integrated PET/MR imaging was deemed impossible. Accordingly, when the first integrated PET/MR imaging entered the market, expectations were very high. It took several years until the first results on cardiovascular applications were published. Now, this modality has proved to be of high relevance not only in a research environment,

but also for certain clinically important indications such as myocardial viability imaging and imaging of focal inflammation of the heart. It is expected that hybrid PET/MR imaging will continue to play a pivotal role in the potential future applications of atherosclerotic plaque imaging and in the assessment and validation of novel cardiovascular imaging biomarkers.

REFERENCES

1. Zaidi H, Ojha N, Morich M, et al. Design and performance evaluation of a whole-body Ingenuity TF PET-MRI system. Phys Med Biol 2011;56:3091–106.
2. Delso G, Furst S, Jakoby B, et al. Performance measurements of the Siemens mMR integrated whole-body PET/MR scanner. J Nucl Med 2011; 52:1914–22.
3. Levin CS, Maramraju SH, Khalighi MM, et al. Design features and mutual compatibility studies of the time-of-flight PET capable GE SIGNA PET/MR system. IEEE Trans Med Imaging 2016;35(8): 1907–14.
4. Pichler BJ, Judenhofer MS, Catana C, et al. Performance test of an LSO-APD detector in a 7-T MRI

scanner for simultaneous PET/MRI. J Nucl Med 2006;47:639–47.

5. Levin C, Deller T, Peterson W, et al. Initial results of simultaneous whole-body ToF PET/MR. J Nucl Med 2014;55(Supplement 1):660, 2014.

6. Huang SC, Carson RE, Phelps ME, et al. A boundary method for attenuation correction in positron computed tomography. J Nucl Med 1981;22:627–37.

7. Coombs BD, Szumowski J, Coshow W. Two-point Dixon technique for water-fat signal decomposition with B0 inhomogeneity correction. Magn Reson Med 1997;38:884–9.

8. Martinez-Moller A, Souvatzoglou M, Delso G, et al. Tissue classification as a potential approach for attenuation correction in whole-body PET/MRI: evaluation with PET/CT data. J Nucl Med 2009; 50:520–6.

9. Schulz V, Torres-Espallardo I, Renisch S, et al. Automatic, three-segment, MR-based attenuation correction for whole-body PET/MR data. Eur J Nucl Med Mol Imaging 2011;38:138–52.

10. Paulus DH, Quick HH, Geppert C, et al. Whole-body PET/MR imaging: quantitative evaluation of a novel model-based MR attenuation correction method including bone. J Nucl Med 2015;56:1061–6.

11. Beyer T, Lassen ML, Boellaard R, et al. Investigating the state-of-the-art in whole-body MR-based attenuation correction: an intra-individual, inter-system, inventory study on three clinical PET/MR systems. MAGMA 2016;29:75–87.

12. Samarin A, Burger C, Wollenweber SD, et al. PET/MR imaging of bone lesions–implications for PET quantification from imperfect attenuation correction. Eur J Nucl Med Mol Imaging 2012;39: 1154–60.

13. Lau JMC, Laforest R, Sotoudeh H, et al. Evaluation of attenuation correction in cardiac PET using PET/MR. J Nucl Cardiol 2017;24:839–46.

14. Nuyts J, Bal G, Kehren F, et al. Completion of a truncated attenuation image from the attenuated PET emission data. IEEE Trans Med Imaging 2013;32(2):237–46.

15. Nuyts J, Dupont P, Stroobants S, et al. Simultaneous maximum a posteriori reconstruction of attenuation and activity distributions from emission sinograms. IEEE Trans Med Imaging 1999;18(5): 393–403.

16. Rischpler C, Nekolla SG, Dregely I, et al. Hybrid PET/MR imaging of the heart: potential, initial experiences, and future prospects. J Nucl Med 2013;54: 402–15.

17. Freitag MT, Fenchel M, Baumer P, et al. Improved clinical workflow for simultaneous whole-body PET/MRI using high-resolution CAIPIRINHA-accelerated MR-based attenuation correction. Eur J Radiol 2017;96:12–20.

18. Jimenez-Ballve A, Perez-Castejon MJ, Delgado-Bolton RC, et al. Assessment of the diagnostic accuracy of (18)F-FDG PET/CT in prosthetic infective endocarditis and cardiac implantable electronic device infection: comparison of different interpretation criteria. Eur J Nucl Med Mol Imaging 2016;43: 2401–12.

19. Lassen ML, Rasul S, Beitzke D, et al. Assessment of attenuation correction for myocardial PET imaging using combined PET/MRI. J Nucl Cardiol 2017. https://doi.org/10.1007/s12350-017-1118-2.

20. Ruhlmann V, Heusch P, Kuhl H, et al. Potential influence of Gadolinium contrast on image segmentation in MR-based attenuation correction with Dixon sequences in whole-body 18F-FDG PET/MR. MAGMA 2016;29:301–8.

21. Fürst S, Souvatzoglu M, Rischpler C, et al. Effects of MR contrast agents on attenuation map generation and cardiac PET quantification in PET/MR. J Nucl Med 2012;53(Supplement 1):139, 2012.

22. Klocke FJ, Baird MG, Lorell BH, et al. ACC/AHA/ ASNC guidelines for the clinical use of cardiac radionuclide imaging–executive summary: a report of the American College of Cardiology/American Heart Association Task Force on practice guidelines (ACC/AHA/ASNC Committee to revise the 1995 guidelines for the clinical use of cardiac radionuclide imaging). J Am Coll Cardiol 2003;42: 1318–33.

23. Yoshinaga K, Chow BJ, Williams K, et al. What is the prognostic value of myocardial perfusion imaging using rubidium-82 positron emission tomography? J Am Coll Cardiol 2006;48:1029–39.

24. Schwaiger M, Melin J. Cardiological applications of nuclear medicine. Lancet 1999;354:661–6.

25. Hachamovitch R, Hayes SW, Friedman JD, et al. Comparison of the short-term survival benefit associated with revascularization compared with medical therapy in patients with no prior coronary artery disease undergoing stress myocardial perfusion single photon emission computed tomography. Circulation 2003;107:2900–7.

26. Merhige ME, Breen WJ, Shelton V, et al. Impact of myocardial perfusion imaging with PET and (82) Rb on downstream invasive procedure utilization, costs, and outcomes in coronary disease management. J Nucl Med 2007;48:1069–76.

27. Flotats A, Bravo PE, Fukushima K, et al. (82)Rb PET myocardial perfusion imaging is superior to (99m) Tc-labelled agent SPECT in patients with known or suspected coronary artery disease. Eur J Nucl Med Mol Imaging 2012;39(8):1233–9.

28. Huisman MC, Higuchi T, Reder S, et al. Initial characterization of an 18F-labeled myocardial perfusion tracer. J Nucl Med 2008;49:630–6.

29. Berman DS, Maddahi J, Tamarappoo BK, et al. Phase II safety and clinical comparison with

single-photon emission computed tomography myocardial perfusion imaging for detection of coronary artery disease: flurpiridaz F 18 positron emission tomography. J Am Coll Cardiol 2013;61: 469–77.

30. Sherif HM, Nekolla SG, Saraste A, et al. Simplified quantification of myocardial flow reserve with flurpiridaz F 18: validation with microspheres in a pig model. J Nucl Med 2011;52:617–24.

31. Rischpler C, Park MJ, Fung GS, et al. Advances in PET myocardial perfusion imaging: F-18 labeled tracers. Ann Nucl Med 2012;26:1–6.

32. Manning WJ, Atkinson DJ, Grossman W, et al. First-pass nuclear magnetic resonance imaging studies using gadolinium-DTPA in patients with coronary artery disease. J Am Coll Cardiol 1991;18:959–65.

33. Nandalur KR, Dwamena BA, Choudhri AF, et al. Diagnostic performance of stress cardiac magnetic resonance imaging in the detection of coronary artery disease: a meta-analysis. J Am Coll Cardiol 2007;50:1343–53.

34. de Jong MC, Genders TS, van Geuns RJ, et al. Diagnostic performance of stress myocardial perfusion imaging for coronary artery disease: a systematic review and meta-analysis. Eur Radiol 2012;22(9):1881–95.

35. Parkash R, deKemp RA, Ruddy TD, et al. Potential utility of rubidium 82 PET quantification in patients with 3-vessel coronary artery disease. J Nucl Cardiol 2004;11:440–9.

36. Kajander SA, Joutsiniemi E, Saraste M, et al. Clinical value of absolute quantification of myocardial perfusion with (15)O-water in coronary artery disease. Circ Cardiovasc Imaging 2011;4:678–84.

37. Schwitter J, Nanz D, Kneifel S, et al. Assessment of myocardial perfusion in coronary artery disease by magnetic resonance: a comparison with positron emission tomography and coronary angiography. Circulation 2001;103:2230–5.

38. Ibrahim T, Nekolla SG, Schreiber K, et al. Assessment of coronary flow reserve: comparison between contrast-enhanced magnetic resonance imaging and positron emission tomography. J Am Coll Cardiol 2002;39:864–70.

39. Jerosch-Herold M. Quantification of myocardial perfusion by cardiovascular magnetic resonance. J Cardiovasc Magn Reson 2010;12:57.

40. Morton G, Chiribiri A, Ishida M, et al. Quantification of absolute myocardial perfusion in patients with coronary artery disease: comparison between cardiovascular magnetic resonance and positron emission tomography. J Am Coll Cardiol 2012;60: 1546–55.

41. Kunze KP, Nekolla SG, Rischpler C, et al. Myocardial perfusion quantification using simultaneously acquired (13) NH3 -ammonia PET and dynamic contrast-enhanced MRI in patients at rest and stress. Magn Reson Med 2018. https://doi.org/10. 1002/mrm.27213.

42. Wissmann L, Gotschy A, Santelli C, et al. Analysis of spatiotemporal fidelity in quantitative 3D first-pass perfusion cardiovascular magnetic resonance. J Cardiovasc Magn Reson 2017;19:11.

43. Hausleiter J, Meyer T, Hermann F, et al. Estimated radiation dose associated with cardiac CT angiography. JAMA 2009;301:500–7.

44. Fink C, Krissak R, Henzler T, et al. Radiation dose at coronary CT angiography: second-generation dual-source CT versus single-source 64-MDCT and first-generation dual-source CT. AJR Am J Roentgenol 2011;196:W550–7.

45. Kim WY, Stuber M, Bornert P, et al. Three-dimensional black-blood cardiac magnetic resonance coronary vessel wall imaging detects positive arterial remodeling in patients with nonsignificant coronary artery disease. Circulation 2002;106:296–9.

46. Fayad ZA, Fuster V, Fallon JT, et al. Noninvasive in vivo human coronary artery lumen and wall imaging using black-blood magnetic resonance imaging. Circulation 2000;102:506–10.

47. Davies JR, Rudd JH, Weissberg PL, et al. Radionuclide imaging for the detection of inflammation in vulnerable plaques. J Am Coll Cardiol 2006;47: C57–68.

48. Rudd JH, Warburton EA, Fryer TD, et al. Imaging atherosclerotic plaque inflammation with [18F]-fluorodeoxyglucose positron emission tomography. Circulation 2002;105:2708–11.

49. Dregely I, Koppara T, Nekolla SG, et al. Observations with simultaneous 18F-FDG PET and MR imaging in peripheral artery disease. JACC Cardiovasc Imaging 2017;10:709–11.

50. Joshi NV, Vesey AT, Williams MC, et al. 18F-fluoride positron emission tomography for identification of ruptured and high-risk coronary atherosclerotic plaques: a prospective clinical trial. Lancet 2014; 383:705–13.

51. Saraste A, Laitinen I, Weidl E, et al. Diet intervention reduces uptake of alphavbeta3 integrin-targeted PET tracer 18F-galacto-RGD in mouse atherosclerotic plaques. J Nucl Cardiol 2012;19: 775–84.

52. Beer AJ, Pelisek J, Heider P, et al. PET/CT imaging of integrin alphavbeta3 expression in human carotid atherosclerosis. JACC Cardiovasc Imaging 2014;7:178–87.

53. Boswijk E, Bauwens M, Mottaghy FM, et al. Potential of alpha7 nicotinic acetylcholine receptor PET imaging in atherosclerosis. Methods 2017;130: 90–104.

54. Hyafil F, Pelisek J, Laitinen I, et al. Imaging the cytokine receptor CXCR4 in atherosclerotic plaques with the radiotracer (68)Ga-pentixafor for PET. J Nucl Med 2017;58:499–506.

55. Weiberg D, Thackeray JT, Daum G, et al. Clinical molecular imaging of chemokine receptor CXCR4 expression in atherosclerotic plaque using (68) Ga-pentixafor PET: correlation with cardiovascular risk factors and calcified plaque burden. J Nucl Med 2018;59:266–72.

56. Li X, Heber D, Leike T, et al. [68Ga]Pentixafor-PET/MRI for the detection of Chemokine receptor 4 expression in atherosclerotic plaques. Eur J Nucl Med Mol Imaging 2018;45:558–66.

57. Derlin T, Sedding DG, Dutzmann J, et al. Imaging of chemokine receptor CXCR4 expression in culprit and nonculprit coronary atherosclerotic plaque using motion-corrected [(68)Ga]pentixafor PET/CT. Eur J Nucl Med Mol Imaging 2018;45(11): 1934–44.

58. Luehmann HP, Pressly ED, Detering L, et al. PET/CT imaging of chemokine receptor CCR5 in vascular injury model using targeted nanoparticle. J Nucl Med 2014;55:629–34.

59. Wei L, Petryk J, Gaudet C, et al. Development of an inflammation imaging tracer, (111)In-DOTA-DAPTA, targeting chemokine receptor CCR5 and preliminary evaluation in an ApoE(-/-) atherosclerosis mouse model. J Nucl Cardiol 2018. https://doi.org/10.1007/s12350-018-1203-1.

60. Liu Y, Woodard PK. Chemokine receptors: key for molecular imaging of inflammation in atherosclerosis. J Nucl Cardiol 2018. https://doi.org/10.1007/s12350-018-1203-1.

61. Zayed MA, Harring SD, Abendschein DR, et al. Natriuretic peptide receptor-C is up-regulated in the intima of advanced carotid artery atherosclerosis. J Med Surg Pathol 2016;1 [pii:131].

62. Liu Y, Abendschein D, Woodard GE, et al. Molecular imaging of atherosclerotic plaque with (64)Cu-labeled natriuretic peptide and PET. J Nucl Med 2010;51:85–91.

63. Liu Y, Pressly ED, Abendschein DR, et al. Targeting angiogenesis using a C-type atrial natriuretic factor-conjugated nanoprobe and PET. J Nucl Med 2011;52:1956–63.

64. Nie X, Randolph GJ, Elvington A, et al. Imaging of hypoxia in mouse atherosclerotic plaques with (64) Cu-ATSM. Nucl Med Biol 2016;43:534–42.

65. Nie X, Laforest R, Elvington A, et al. PET/MRI of hypoxic atherosclerosis using 64Cu-ATSM in a rabbit model. J Nucl Med 2016;57:2006–11.

66. Munoz C, Kunze KP, Neji R, et al. Motion-corrected whole-heart PET-MR for the simultaneous visualisation of coronary artery integrity and myocardial viability: an initial clinical validation. Eur J Nucl Med Mol Imaging 2018;45:1975–86.

67. Ghosh N, Rimoldi OE, Beanlands RS, et al. Assessment of myocardial ischaemia and viability: role of positron emission tomography. Eur Heart J 2010; 31:2984–95.

68. Di Carli MF. Predicting improved function after myocardial revascularization. Curr Opin Cardiol 1998;13:415–24.

69. Beanlands RS, Hendry PJ, Masters RG, et al. Delay in revascularization is associated with increased mortality rate in patients with severe left ventricular dysfunction and viable myocardium on fluorine 18-fluorodeoxyglucose positron emission tomography imaging. Circulation 1998;98:II51–6.

70. Di Carli MF, Davidson M, Little R, et al. Value of metabolic imaging with positron emission tomography for evaluating prognosis in patients with coronary artery disease and left ventricular dysfunction. Am J Cardiol 1994;73:527–33.

71. D'Egidio G, Nichol G, Williams KA, et al. Increasing benefit from revascularization is associated with increasing amounts of myocardial hibernation: a substudy of the PARR-2 trial. JACC Cardiovasc Imaging 2009;2:1060–8.

72. Allman KC, Shaw LJ, Hachamovitch R, et al. Myocardial viability testing and impact of revascularization on prognosis in patients with coronary artery disease and left ventricular dysfunction: a meta-analysis. J Am Coll Cardiol 2002;39: 1151–8.

73. Klein C, Nekolla SG, Bengel FM, et al. Assessment of myocardial viability with contrast-enhanced magnetic resonance imaging: comparison with positron emission tomography. Circulation 2002; 105:162–7.

74. Kim RJ, Wu E, Rafael A, et al. The use of contrast-enhanced magnetic resonance imaging to identify reversible myocardial dysfunction. N Engl J Med 2000;343:1445–53.

75. Kwong RY, Chan AK, Brown KA, et al. Impact of unrecognized myocardial scar detected by cardiac magnetic resonance imaging on event-free survival in patients presenting with signs or symptoms of coronary artery disease. Circulation 2006;113: 2733–43.

76. Schinkel AF, Bax JJ, Poldermans D, et al. Hibernating myocardium: diagnosis and patient outcomes. Curr Probl Cardiol 2007;32:375–410.

77. Rischpler C, Langwieser N, Souvatzoglou M, et al. PET/MRI early after myocardial infarction: evaluation of viability with late gadolinium enhancement transmurality vs. 18F-FDG uptake. Eur Heart J Cardiovasc Imaging 2015;16:661–9.

78. Priamo J, Adamopoulos D, Rager O, et al. Downstream indication to revascularization following hybrid cardiac PET/MRI: preliminary results. Nucl Med Commun 2017;38:515–22.

79. Nensa F, Poeppel TD, Beiderwellen K, et al. Hybrid PET/MR imaging of the heart: feasibility and initial results. Radiology 2013;268:366–73.

80. Nensa F, Poeppel T, Tezgah E, et al. Integrated FDG PET/MR imaging for the assessment of

myocardial salvage in reperfused acute myocardial infarction. Radiology 2015;276:400–7.

81. Heusch P, Nensa F, Heusch G. Is MRI really the gold standard for the quantification of salvage from myocardial infarction? Circ Res 2015;117:222–4.

82. Erba PA, Sollini M, Lazzeri E, et al. FDG-PET in cardiac infections. Semin Nucl Med 2013;43:377–95.

83. Nensa F, Tezgah E, Schweins K, et al. Evaluation of a low-carbohydrate diet-based preparation protocol without fasting for cardiac PET/MR imaging. J Nucl Cardiol 2017;24:980–8.

84. Scholtens AM, Verberne HJ, Budde RP, et al. Additional heparin preadministration improves cardiac glucose metabolism suppression over low-carbohydrate diet alone in 18F-FDG PET imaging. J Nucl Med 2016;57:568–73.

85. Rischpler C, Nekolla SG, Kossmann H, et al. Upregulated myocardial CXCR4-expression after myocardial infarction assessed by simultaneous GA-68 pentixafor PET/MRI. J Nucl Cardiol 2016;23:131–3.

86. Nensa F, Poeppel TD, Krings P, et al. Multiparametric assessment of myocarditis using simultaneous positron emission tomography/magnetic resonance imaging. Eur Heart J 2014;35:2173.

87. von Olshausen G, Hyafil F, Langwieser N, et al. Detection of acute inflammatory myocarditis in Epstein Barr virus infection using hybrid 18F-fluorodeoxyglucose-positron emission tomography/magnetic resonance imaging. Circulation 2014;130:925–6.

88. Piriou N, Sassier J, Pallardy A, et al. Utility of cardiac FDG-PET imaging coupled to magnetic resonance for the management of an acute myocarditis with non-informative endomyocardial biopsy. Eur Heart J Cardiovasc Imaging 2015;16:574.

89. Nensa F, Kloth J, Tezgah E, et al. Feasibility of FDG-PET in myocarditis: comparison to CMR using integrated PET/MRI. J Nucl Cardiol 2018;25:785–94.

90. Friedrich MG, Sechtem U, Schulz-Menger J, et al. Cardiovascular magnetic resonance in myocarditis: a JACC white paper. J Am Coll Cardiol 2009;53:1475–87.

91. Sekiguchi M, Numao Y, Imai M, et al. Clinical and histopathological profile of sarcoidosis of the heart and acute idiopathic myocarditis. Concepts through a study employing endomyocardial biopsy. I. Sarcoidosis. Jpn Circ J 1980;44:249–63.

92. Birnie DH, Sauer WH, Bogun F, et al. HRS expert consensus statement on the diagnosis and management of arrhythmias associated with cardiac sarcoidosis. Heart Rhythm 2014;11:1305–23.

93. Blankstein R, Osborne M, Naya M, et al. Cardiac positron emission tomography enhances prognostic assessments of patients with suspected cardiac sarcoidosis. J Am Coll Cardiol 2014;63:329–36.

94. Schneider S, Batrice A, Rischpler C, et al. Utility of multimodal cardiac imaging with PET/MRI in cardiac sarcoidosis: implications for diagnosis, monitoring and treatment. Eur Heart J 2014;35:312.

95. Wada K, Niitsuma T, Yamaki T, et al. Simultaneous cardiac imaging to detect inflammation and scar tissue with (18)F-fluorodeoxyglucose PET/MRI in cardiac sarcoidosis. J Nucl Cardiol 2016;23:1180–2.

96. Hanneman K, Kadoch M, Guo HH, et al. Initial experience with simultaneous 18F-FDG PET/MRI in the evaluation of cardiac sarcoidosis and myocarditis. Clin Nucl Med 2017;42:e328–34.

97. Kiko T, Masuda A, Nemoto A, et al. Cardiac sarcoidosis after glucocorticoid therapy evaluated by (18)F-fluorodeoxyglucose PET/MRI. J Nucl Cardiol 2018;25:685–7.

98. van der Laan AM, Nahrendorf M, Piek JJ. Healing and adverse remodelling after acute myocardial infarction: role of the cellular immune response. Heart 2012;98:1384–90.

99. Curley D, Lavin Plaza B, Shah AM, et al. Molecular imaging of cardiac remodelling after myocardial infarction. Basic Res Cardiol 2018;113:10.

100. Heusch G, Libby P, Gersh B, et al. Cardiovascular remodelling in coronary artery disease and heart failure. Lancet 2014;383:1933–43.

101. Lee WW, Marinelli B, van der Laan AM, et al. PET/MRI of inflammation in myocardial infarction. J Am Coll Cardiol 2012;59:153–63.

102. Wollenweber T, Roentgen P, Schafer A, et al. Characterizing the inflammatory tissue response to acute myocardial infarction by clinical multimodality noninvasive imaging. Circ Cardiovasc Imaging 2014;7:811–8.

103. Rischpler C, Dirschinger RJ, Nekolla SG, et al. Prospective evaluation of 18F-fluorodeoxyglucose uptake in postischemic myocardium by simultaneous positron emission tomography/magnetic resonance imaging as a prognostic marker of functional outcome. Circ Cardiovasc Imaging 2016;9:e004316.

The Potential Role of Total Body PET Imaging in Assessment of Atherosclerosis

Jeffrey P. Schmall, PhD*, Joel S. Karp, PhD,
Abass Alavi, MD, MD (Hon), PhD (Hon), DSc (Hon)

KEYWORDS

- Atherosclerosis - PET imaging - Total body PET imaging - Cardiovascular disorders
- Plaque burden

KEY POINTS

- Advances in molecular imaging along with PET instrumentation will be of great value in assessing atherosclerosis plaques, and potentially other cardiovascular disorders.
- Atherosclerosis is systemic and involves critical arteries including carotids, coronaries and peripheral vessels.
- Total body PET imaging will allow assessment of disease throughout the body and monitoring of the course throughout therapeutic interventions.
- The high sensitivity of total body PET instruments permits generation of data with robust statistical properties, which we expect will be used for delayed imaging of F18 NaF and F18 FDG in the assessment of atherosclerosis.

IMAGING TECHNIQUES APPLIED TO ATHEROSCLEROSIS

Atherosclerosis (AS) is a common cause of morbidity and mortality in the aging population worldwide. It is estimated that 10 million people succumb to complications of AS plaques, namely, heart attacks and strokes, per year, despite advances in prevention and treatment.[1,2] Clinical evaluations and invasive procedures such as contrast-enhanced angiography are of limited value for the diagnosis and monitoring of response to treatment.[3] The introduction of computed tomography (CT) in the 1970s has allowed for the detection and characterization of calcification in the coronary and major arteries.[4] However, using CT scans to assess calcification in the vasculature is of limited value in optimal management of patients. This is due to the fact that calcification detected by CT scans represents an advanced phase of this

process and is irreversible with current treatments. In recent years, with advances in CT imaging, it is feasible to perform noninvasive angiography of the coronary arteries with significant detail.[5] By now it is well-established that structural changes, including narrowing of the arterial lumen by the atherosclerotic disease or calcification, are unable to predict plaque rupture and, therefore, thrombosis in the affected vessels.[6–8] Thus, there is a need for newer technologies that can detect vulnerable plaques in the early phase of the disease and prevent serious complications associated with the evolution of the underlying process.

During the past few decades, molecular imaging techniques that allow for the visualization of preliminary stages and microscopic evidence of many disorders have been introduced.[9] If this approach is validated in animal and human studies of AS, the impact will be substantial in preventing complications of this disorder. It is known that

Department of Radiology, University of Pennsylvania, 3620 Hamilton Walk, 1st Floor John Morgan Building, Philadelphia, PA 19104, USA
* Corresponding author. 3400 Civic Center Boulevard, Philadelphia, PA 19104.
E-mail address: schmall@pennmedicine.upenn.edu

PET Clin 14 (2019) 245–250
https://doi.org/10.1016/j.cpet.2018.12.007
1556-8598/19/© 2018 Elsevier Inc. All rights reserved.

molecular changes are the earliest biomarker for a number of benign and malignant disorders,[10] and these molecular signals are well-measured using PET. Molecular disease eventually leads to functional abnormalities, such as change in blood flow to the organs affected. Structural abnormalities follow the functional changes; therefore, when anatomic changes are detected by CT scans or MRI, the disease process is irreversible and leads to serious consequences.

In recent years, PET imaging with fludeoxyglucose F 18 (^{18}F FDG) and sodium fluoride F 18 ([18]F NaF) has been widely tested for the detection and characterization of AS plaques in the coronaries and major arteries.[11] [18]F FDG is known to visualize inflammatory cells and is being used for the detection of disease activity in the lungs, infections, and joint diseases.[12] Therefore, ^{18}F FDG PET imaging allows for the detection of atherosclerotic plaques that contain a large number of macrophages in the active phase of the disease.[11,13] In contrast, PET imaging with [18]F NaF visualizes molecular calcification in the plaques.[11] Recent data show greater sensitivity for molecular calcification by [18]F NaF compared with that of ^{18}F FDG PET imaging for inflammation.[13] Therefore, based on these data, it is foreseeable that [18]F NaF imaging to detect molecular calcification may become the technique of choice to monitor the course of AS. In addition, it has become apparent that global disease assessment is superior to measurements at the regional level for the quantification of AS burden in the arteries.[14]

RECENT ADVANCES IN PET INSTRUMENTATION

Concurrently, directly relevant to PET imaging of AS are major technological advancements in PET instrumentation, which have enabled new PET instruments capable of measuring the tracer distribution in the whole body simultaneously—referred to as total body PET (TB PET)—rather than the fusion of images from multiple bed positions as is done with current clinical PET instruments.[15] TB PET instruments have the same ring design as conventional PET instruments, with a ring diameter in the range of approximately 70 to 80 cm, creating a transverse imaging field of view (FOV) that approximately 50 to 60 cm, but have an elongated axial imaging FOV—as long as approximately 200 cm compared with approximately 20 cm available with current PET designs, such that the entire body is surrounded by detectors (**Fig. 1**). Because the entire body is within the imaging FOV, the tracer uptake from all organs and tissues can be quantified simultaneously with good temporal resolution. Although concepts of TB PET were originally proposed decades ago, the current development is primarily a result of the Explorer PET program[16]; the motivation, preliminary studies, and progress has been discussed in several recent reviews.[17–19] To understand how TB PET will impact cardiovascular imaging of AS, we first provide some basic background of the underlying physics principles motivating TB PET and then discuss some specific directions for imaging AS using TB PET instruments.

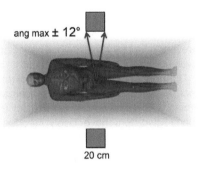

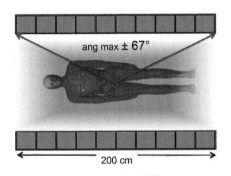

ang max ± 12°

20 cm

Standard whole-body PET

ang max ± 67°

200 cm

Total-body PET

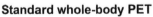

Fig. 1. The total body (TB) PET instrument concept. By having the patient surrounded by detectors the entire body can be imaged simultaneously with no movement of the imaging bed. A second advantage of TB PET is the wider axial acceptance angle (shown as ang max), which further increases photon sensitivity by capturing oblique photons that cannot be detected with standard 20-cm PET. The increased photon attenuation through the body limits photon sensitivity gains for very wide acceptance angles,[20] and therefore the greatest usefulness of a TB PET instrument will be for imaging applications of the whole body rather than applications focused on a single organ or limited patient coverage.

CONCEPT OF TOTAL BODY PET

The photon signal (from positron–electron annihilation) is isotropic; therefore, the amount of signal captured by the PET scanner can be quantified by calculating the solid angle coverage. Depending on the imaging application the source distribution (ie, patient coverage) will change. For example, imaging applications where the entire body needs to be scanned results in a very low solid angle coverage when using current approximately 20 cm axial FOV instruments because most of the patient is outside of the imaging FOV for a given bed position; if the imaging study is only focused on a single organ (the heart or the brain), the solid angle coverage is much better. The comparison that is often made is to relate the photon sensitivity (number of events detected by the PET system) of a 20-cm-long scanner (current apparent FOV PET) with that of a 200-cm scanner (TB PET); based on the argument regarding source distribution and solid angle coverage, estimates of the gain in photon sensitivity with TB PET are approximately 4× for a single organ, and up to an approximately 40× gain can be achieved for whole body imaging applications. These estimates for the 2-m system were based on computer simulations[21,22]; however, currently 2 long axial FOV PET scanners have been constructed and experimental measurements have confirmed many of these predicted gains in photon sensitivity[23,24] (**Fig. 2**). The main question that now remains is how to use these TB PET instruments effectively and evaluate their impact on current clinical applications and research studies, more specifically in the assessment of AS, as described herein.

The predicted 40× gain in whole body photon sensitivity with TB PET can be used in a variety of ways for cardiovascular imaging. An obvious approach to use this gain in photon sensitivity would be to inject 1/40 of the radiotracer activity, resulting in scans with 1/40 of the radiation dose. Another approach would be to scan for 1/40 of the time, acquiring whole body scans in as little as approximately 30 seconds. There are many other ways to use such a pronounced gain in sensitivity, such as enabling reconstructions at higher resolution to decrease partial volume effects and detect smaller lesions with lower contrast, or to better use kinetic modeling techniques with high temporal resolution by taking advantage of the better count statistics offered by high sensitivity, and potentially many more approaches, some of which have not yet been conceived.

TOTAL BODY PET FOR IMAGING ATHEROSCLEROSIS

For applications in AS plaque imaging with TB PET, we hypothesize that delayed imaging will be a primary application. Both ^{18}F NaF and ^{18}F FDG have been shown to benefit from long uptake times and delayed image acquisition, because the tracer contrast generally improves with time[25,26]; however, with current PET instruments the trade off from delayed images with improved contrast is of course images with less counts and therefore greater noise. Theoretically, a 40× gain in sensitivity with TB PET would allow ^{18}F tracers (injected with the same dose) to be imaged out to 5 half-lives (a 10-hour uptake time) with the same noise characteristics as scans on current PET instruments using a standard 1-hour

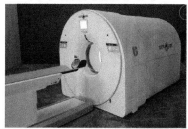

UIH Explorer
194 cm Axial FOV

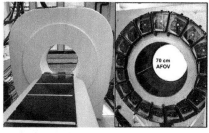

PennPET Explorer
70 cm Axial FOV

Fig. 2. The 2 prototype long-axial PET systems currently constructed as part of the Explorer consortium. (LEFT) A commercially built total body PET/CT scanner from (United Imaging, Shanghai, China) that provides total body coverage with high spatial resolution detectors. (*Right*) A 70-cm system developed at the University of Pennsylvania that allows for complete torso imaging using detectors with advanced time-of-flight capability. This scanner design is scalable and there are plans to expand beyond 70-cm axial field of view. (*From* Cherry SR, Jones T, Karp JS, et al: Total-body PET: maximizing sensitivity to create new opportunities for clinical research and patient care. J Nucl Med 2018;59:3–12.)

uptake time. Recent studies suggest that the optimal uptake time for AS imaging with [18]F NaF, as well as ^{18}F FDG, would be in the range of 3 to 4 hours.[27] Delayed whole body images with uptake times extended from 1 hour (current) to 3 hours (delayed) would only represent an approximately a one-half decrease (53%) in tracer activity, and therefore imaging protocols with a TB PET scanner could allow for significant reductions in either dose or scan time (or a combination of both), as well as delayed acquisition. Techniques for cardiac gating or respiratory gating also become feasible and have the potential to significantly improve resolution with little to no increase in noise owing to the high system sensitivity. Low-dose, delayed imaging scans could also be very advantageous for imaging applications that measure response to AS therapies—unlike most other diseases, there are several drugs that are very effective at treating AS,[28,29] and with low-dose imaging techniques, repeated monitoring with PET could become an effective strategy for patient management without cumulative absorbed dose concerns.

Last, symptoms of AS disease involve the entire body and often present as a systemic disease. Therefore, total body imaging will allow optimal assessment of disease activity and progression with higher accuracy and precision compared with conventional imaging techniques because the instrument is specifically designed to have whole body coverage, enabling dynamic measurement of the vascular system throughout the body and the interplay of multiorgan processes.

SUMMARY

It is clear that recent advances made in molecular imaging along with PET instrumentation will be of great value in assessing AS plaques, and potentially other cardiovascular disorders. AS is systemic in nature and involves critical arteries including carotids, coronaries and peripheral vessels. TB PET imaging will allow assessment of the disease throughout the body and monitoring of the course throughout therapeutic interventions. The high sensitivity of TB PET instruments (>40-fold compared with conventional PET instruments) will permit generation of data with robust statistical properties, that is, these images provide more than a 6-fold increase in signal-to-noise ratio compared with current state of the art scanners. Because of the high sensitivity of TB PET, delayed imaging can be performed hours after the administration of the tracer compounds of interest. This

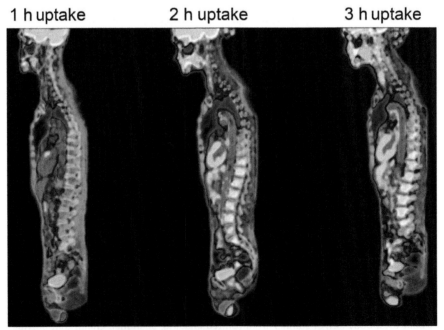

Fig. 3. A sagittal fludeoxyglucose F 18 (^{18}F FDG) PET image of the thoracic aorta illustrates changes in aortic wall and blood pool ^{18}F FDG activity at different imaging time points. The arterial wall-to-blood contrast improves over time, because the blood pool activity decreases and the aortic wall activity increases, and this results in a superior target-to-background ratio. A TB PET instrument will provide better image quality, for a fixed imaging time, at late time points owing to the higher system photon sensitivity.

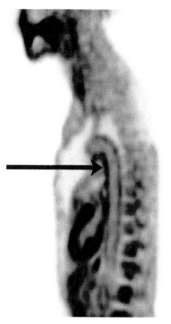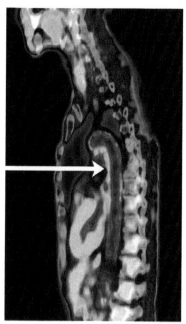

Fig. 4. The PET image on the left reveals significant uptake of ^{18}F FDG in the thoracic aorta without anatomic landmarks, whereas the PET/computed tomography (CT) image on the right demonstrates the exact location of ^{18}F FDG uptake in various structures, including atherosclerotic plaques. PET-CT imaging has become the standard ever since it was introduced in 2001. This combination significantly enhances the impact of PET imaging for patient care and research studies with this powerful modality. The engineering challenges associated with the integration of CT with TB PET are still on going, but are expected to provide integrated TB PET/CT imaging systems.

strategy results in higher contrast at the disease site compared with background (**Figs. 3** and **4**). This information is of great importance in assessing AS plaques in the arteries. Also, a global assessment of the plaque burden throughout the body including the coronary arteries will substantially improve our ability to quantify plaque activity in the course of the disease.

ACKNOWLEDGMENTS

This work was funded by the National Institute of Health through grants R01CA113941 and R01CA206187. The content is solely the responsibility of the authors and does not necessarily represent the official views of the National Institutes of Health.

REFERENCES

1. Lloyd-Jones D, Adams R, Carnethon M, et al. Heart disease and stroke statistics—2009 update: a report from the American Heart Association Statistics Committee and Stroke Statistics Subcommittee. Circulation 2009;119(3):e21–181.
2. Lozano R, Naghavi M, Foreman K, et al. Global and regional mortality from 235 causes of death for 20 age groups in 1990 and 2010: a systematic analysis for the Global Burden of Disease Study 2010. Lancet 2012;380(9859):2095–128.
3. Wilms G, Baert AL. The history of angiography. J Belge Radiol 1995;78(5):299–302.
4. Agatston AS, Janowitz WR, Hildner FJ, et al. Quantification of coronary artery calcium using ultra- fast computed tomography. J Am Coll Cardiol 1990; 15(4):827–32.
5. Willemink MJ. Coronary artery calcium: a technical argument for a new scoring method. J Cardiovasc Comput Tomogr 2018. https://doi.org/10.1016/j.jcct. 2018.
6. Alavi A, Werner TJ, Høilund-Carlsen PF. PET-based imaging to detect and characterize cardiovascular disorders: unavoidable path for the foreseeable future. J Nucl Cardiol 2018;25:203.
7. Alavi A, Werner TJ, Høilund-Carlsen PF. What can be and what cannot be accomplished with PET to detect and characterize atherosclerotic plaques. J Nucl Cardiol 2017. https://doi.org/10.1007/s12350-017-0977-x.
8. Moghbel M, Al-Zaghal A, Werner TJ, et al. The role of PET in evaluating atherosclerosis: a critical review. Semin Nucl Med 2018;48(6):488–97.
9. Hess S, Blomberg BA, Zhu HJ, et al. The pivotal role of FDG-PET/CT in modern medicine. Acad Radiol 2014;21(2):232–49.

10. Alavi A, Werner TJ, Høilund-Carlsen PF. What can be and what cannot be accomplished with PET: rectifying ongoing misconceptions. Clin Nucl Med 2017;42(8):603–5.

11. McKenney-Drake ML, Moghbel MC, Paydary K, et al. 18F-NaF and 18F-FDG as molecular probes in the evaluation of atherosclerosis. Eur J Nucl Med Mol Imaging 2018;45(12):2190–200.

12. Al-Zaghal A, Raynor W, Khosravi M, et al. Applications of PET imaging in the evaluation of musculo-skeletal diseases among the geriatric population. Semin Nucl Med 2018;48(6):525–34.

13. Bloomberg BA, De Jong PA, Thomassen A, et al. Thoracic aorta calcification but not inflammation is associated with increased cardiovascular disease risk: results of the CAMONA study. Eur J Nucl Med Mol Imaging 2017;44(2):249–58.

14. Bloomberg BA, Thomassen A, De Jong PA, et al. Reference values for fluorine-18-fluorodeoxyglucose and fluorine-18-sodium fluoride uptake in human arteries: a prospective evaluation of 89 healthy adults. Nucl Med Commun 2017;38(11):998–1006.

15. Berg E, Cherry SR. Innovation in instrumentation for positron emission tomography. Semin Nucl Med 2018;48(4).

16. University of California Davis. Explorer. Available at: https://explorer.ucdavis.edu/.

17. Cherry SR, Badawi RD, Karp JS, et al. Total-body imaging: transforming the role of positron emission tomography. Sci Transl Med 2017;9(381) [pii: eaaf6169].

18. Cherry SR, Jones T, Karp JS, et al. Total-body PET: maximizing sensitivity to create new opportunities for clinical research and patient care. J Nucl Med 2018;59:3–12.

19. Viswanath V, Daube-Witherspoon ME, Schmall JP, et al. Development of PET for total-body imaging. Acta Phys Pol B 2017;48(10).

20. Schmall JP, Karp JS, Werner M, et al. Parallax error in long-axial field-of-view PET scanners—a simulation study. Phys Med Biol 2016;61(14):5443–55.

21. Poon JK, Dahlbom ML, Moses WW, et al. Optimal whole-body PET scanner configurations for different volumes of LSO scintillator: a simulation study. Phys Med Biol 2012;57(13):4077.

22. Zhang X, Zhou J, Cherry SR, et al. Quantitative image reconstruction for total-body PET imaging using the 2-meter long EXPLORER scanner. Phys Med Biol 2017;62(6):2465.

23. Badawi R, Liu W, Berg E, et al. Progress on the EXPLORER project: towards a total body PET scanner for human imaging. J Nucl Med 2018;59(supplement 1):223.

24. Karp J, Schmall J, Geagan M, et al. Imaging performance of the PennPET explorer scanner. J Nucl Med 2018;59(supplement 1):222.

25. Blomberg BA, Thomassen A, Takx RAP, et al. Delayed 18F- fluorodeoxyglucose PET/CT imaging improves quantitation of atherosclerotic plaque inflammation: results from the CAMONA study. J Nucl Cardiol 2014;21:588–97.

26. Blomberg BA, Thomassen A, Takx RA, et al. Delayed sodium 18 F-fluoride PET/CT imaging does not improve quantification of vascular calcification metabolism: results from the CAMONA study. J Nucl Cardiol 2014;21(2):293–304.

27. Kwiecinski J, Berman DS, Lee SE, et al. Three-hour delayed imaging improves assessment of coronary 18F-sodium fluoride PET. J Nucl Med 2018. [Epub ahead of print].

28. Solanki A, Bhatt LK, Thomas P, et al. Evolving targets for the treatment of atherosclerosis. Pharmacology & therapeutics 2018;187:1–12.

29. Bäck M, Hansson GK. Anti-inflammatory therapies for atherosclerosis. Nat Rev Cardiol 2015;12(4):199.

PET/Computed Tomography Evaluation of Infection of the Heart

Beverley Cherie Millar, PhD[a],*,
Raphael Abegão de Camargo, MD, PhD[b,c],
Abass Alavi, MD, MD (Hon), PhD (Hon), DSc (Hon)[d],
John Edmund Moore, PhD[a]

KEYWORDS

- Cardiac device • Endocarditis • Graft infection • Infection • Left ventricular assist device
- Pacemaker • PET

KEY POINTS

- Background relating to cardiac infections, current diagnosis and limitations, international guidelines.
- The role of ^{18}F-fluorodeoxyglucose (^{18}F-FDG)-PET/computed tomography (CT) in the diagnosis and monitoring of secondary complications associated with infective endocarditis, cardiac implantable device infection, left ventricular assist device infection and graft infection.
- Current limitations in the use of ^{18}F-FDG-PET/CT to diagnose and monitor cardiac infection.
- Current best-practice protocols.

INTRODUCTION

Cardiac infections are predominantly endocardial, namely infective endocarditis (IE), attributed to native or prosthetic heart valves, as well as infection associated with indwelling cardiac implantable electronic devices (CIEDs), such as pacemakers, cardioverters, and left ventricular assist devices (LVADs).[1,2] In addition, cardiac infection may be attributed to infective myocarditis, pericarditis, or recent cardiac surgery, including prosthetic aortic grafts.[1–3] The diagnosis of these infections may be difficult; therefore, clinical presentation and microbiological and enhanced imaging approaches have been used to aid in reaching a definitive and accurate diagnosis.

INFECTIVE ENDOCARDITIS: CURRENT DIAGNOSTIC APPROACHES

Because of the underlying risk factors, varied causative infectious agents, and associated secondary complications of IE, the diagnosis, clinical management, and monitoring of IE require a multidisciplinary approach.[4,5] The initial diagnosis is a challenge, because of a myriad of clinical presentations, many of which are nonspecific to IE. The Modified Duke Criteria have offered guidance and have become an international diagnostic cornerstone, with major criteria focusing on microbiological evidence, namely positive blood culture, positive serology for *Coxiella burnetii*, and evidence of endocardial involvement on echocardiography.[6]

Disclosure: None.
[a] Northern Ireland Public Health Laboratory, Department of Bacteriology, Corry Building, Belfast City Hospital, Lisburn Road, Belfast, Co. Antrim BT9 7AD, Northern Ireland, UK; [b] Nuclear Medicine and Infectious Diseases, University of Sao Paulo Medical School (FMUSP), Sao Paulo, Sao Paulo, Brazil; [c] Hospital Aristides Maltez, Avenida Dom João VI, n° 332, Serviço de Medicina Nuclear, 2° subssolo, Brotas, CEP: 40285-001, Salvador-BA, Brazil; [d] Division of Nuclear Medicine, Department of Radiology, Hospital of the University of Pennsylvania, 110 Donner Building, 3400 Spruce Street, Philadelphia, PA 19104, USA
* Corresponding author.
E-mail address: bcmillar@niphl.dnet.co.uk

Echocardiography is central to the diagnosis and management of patients with IE, with evidence of an oscillating intracardiac mass or vegetation, an annular abscess, prosthetic valve partial dehiscence and new valvular regurgitation classified as major criteria in the diagnosis of IE.[6,7] In addition, echocardiography is useful in the prognostic assessment of patients with IE after therapy as well as during and after surgery.[4] The sensitivity for the diagnosis of vegetations in native and prosthetic valves is superior for transesophageal echocardiography (TEE) compared with transthoracic echocardiography (TTE); 96% and 92% versus 70% and 50%, respectively, with specificity around 90% for both TTE and TEE.[4] In general, TTE is performed initially in all cases of suspected IE, with TEE used in cases in which the initial TTE images are negative but there is a strong suspicion of IE or if there is concern for intracardiac complications with an initial positive TTE.[4]

The Modified Duke Criteria are specific and sensitive and diagnose approximately 80% of cases of IE; however, there are situations in which the criteria are not fulfilled but there is a strong clinical suspension of IE. Culture-negative microbiological findings may result from fastidious causal organisms, prior antimicrobial therapy, or location of vegetations. The identification of causal agents is fundamental in ensuring that appropriate antimicrobial therapy is both timely and appropriate. Molecular approaches using polymerase chain reaction (PCR), particularly in cases of culture-negative IE, have proved useful, with the suggestion that a molecular diagnosis should be included in the Duke classification scheme.[5,8,9] Furthermore, when real-time PCR is used, an earlier result is obtainable compared with the conventional blood culture.[10] As such, the European Society of Cardiology (ESC) IE diagnostic guidelines include PCR amplification of microbial DNA from heart valve tissue and/or blood samples in cases of culture-negative IE.[4]

Echographic evidence may be inconclusive or difficult to interpret, particularly in the case of small vegetations, coexisting other cardiac changes (eg, degenerative lesions, pseudoaneurysms), or in patients with prosthetic heart valves or intracardiac devices. Additional imaging modalities, such as cardiac computed tomography (CT), magnetic resonance imaging (MRI), and ^{18}F-fluorodeoxyglucose ^{18}F-FDG PET/CT are therefore being investigated in conjunction with echocardiography, each of which have their own advantages and limitations, which are summarized in **Table 1**. At present, although the American Heart Association (AHA) acknowledges the potential of these modalities, until the current limitations/risks and benefits are more fully defined, they have not made any recommendations on their use in relation to the diagnosis of IE.[7] In contrast, the ESC advocates the use of not only TTE and TEE but also multislice CT, PET-MRI, and nuclear imaging in the diagnosis of IE and secondary complications.[4] Furthermore, the ESC guideline acknowledges that nuclear imaging modalities such as single-photon emission CT (SPECT)/CT and ^{18}F-FDG-PET/CT have the potential to reduce the rate of misdiagnosed cases of IE, classified in the possible IE category using the Modified Duke Criteria, as well as detection of peripheral embolic and metastatic infectious events. In light of the potential adjuvant role offered by these imaging modalities in the diagnosis of IE, the ESC has modified the Duke Criteria to include specific details relating to such enhanced imaging findings (**Table 2**).[4]

Following publication of the AHA and ESC guidelines in 2015, there has been an extensive international contribution in the literature relating specifically to the potential role of ^{18}F-FDG-PET/CT in the diagnostic approach to cardiac infection. This article therefore examines the literature from the last 3 years to highlight the additional role ^{18}F-FDG-PET/CT can contribute to an accurate diagnosis of cardiac infections and associated infectious complications. The challenges and pitfalls associated with ^{18}F-FDG-PET/CT in such clinical settings must be recognized and these are discussed along with the suggested protocols that may be incorporated in an attempt to address these issues.

PROSTHETIC VALVE ENDOCARDITIS

The application of ^{18}F-FDG-PET/CT in relation to IE is most recognized and accepted in the diagnostic work-up of prosthetic valve endocarditis (PVE), as shown by its inclusion in the ESC guidelines, where there is a high level of clinical suspicion in patients with prosthetic valves and when the diagnosis is classified as possible or rejected, even following repeat microbiology and TTE[4] (**Fig. 1**). Subsequently, this was supported by the findings of a best-evidence analysis of observational studies.[11] More recently, a large-scale prospective study of 224 episodes of suspected endocarditis (124 PVE and 88 native valve endocarditis [NVE]) reported an improved diagnostic sensitivity, when ^{18}F-FDG-PET/CT was combined with the Modified Duke Criteria on admission (sensitivity, specificity, positive and negative predictive values: 95%, 90%, 91%, and 95%, respectively).[12] Furthermore, in cases of PVE, including abnormal ^{18}F-FDG cardiac uptake as a new major criterion at admission for initial diagnoses enabled recategorization of 91% (29 out of 32) of cases

Table 1
Use of cardiac imaging to aid in the diagnosis of cardiac-related infections as per published studies

	Echocardiography	CT	PET-MRI	PET/CT and PET/CTA	Leukocyte Scintigraphy with SPECT or SPECT/CT
Indications for Use from Published Studies	TTE/TEE • Diagnosis of IE • Prognostic assessment • Perioperative evaluation • Therapeutic evaluation • Embolic risk assessment • Sensitivity PVE: TTE 50%; TEE 92% NVE: TTE 75%; TEE 96% • Easy to use • Highly validated • Broad availability • Universally accepted in international guidelines	Multislice CT • Diagnosis of NVE, PVE, perivalvular lesions, prostheses-related vegetations, abscesses, pseudoaneurysms • Accuracy similar to TEE, possibly superior in terms of extent and consequences of any perivalvular extension; eg, anatomy of pseudoaneurysms, abscesses, and fistulae • Useful in cases involving calcified valves • Detection of emboli/silent emboli, intra-abdominal abscesses, CNS lesions • High temporal and special resolution • Quick (minutes) Coronary CTA • Coronary artery evaluation of patients before cardiac surgery for IE complications	• Accurate and superior sensitivity to CT in the diagnosis of neurologic complications, particularly those that are clinically silent • Detection of emboli • Diagnosis of vertebral osteomyelitis	• Early diagnosis of PVE • Doubtful cases of IE • Assessment of emboli and metastatic complications • LVAD driveline infection • Noninvasive • Inclusion in ESC guidelines for diagnosis of PVE and secondary complications	• Diagnosis of PVE and CIED infection • Higher specificity than PET • Discrimination between infection and inflammation • Can be used during first 2 mo postoperatively

(continued on next page)

Table 1
(continued)

	Echocardiography	CT	PET-MRI	PET/CT and PET/CTA	Leukocyte Scintigraphy with SPECT or SPECT/CT
Pitfalls	• False-negative/false-positive • Diagnosis and postoperative evaluation of CIED infection difficult • Late diagnosis	• Routine use not recommended • TEE superior in cases with small vegetations or valve perforation • Limited data • Requires experience • Lack of availability • Use of iodine contrast not advocated in some patients because of nephrotoxicity	• Lower spatial resolution than multislice CT • Lack of availability • Time consuming • Limited use in CIED infection	• Limited large-scale studies • Physiologic uptake of tracer in cardiac tissue • Lack standardization and interpretation experience • Limited availability • Not advocated in unstable patients • Cost • False-positives (surgical glue) • Limited value in diagnosis of NVE and LVAD pump housing infection	• Longer acquisition times than PET • Lower sensitivity than PET • Highly specialized equipment requirement • Safety risks associated with handling patients' blood • Use heavy isotope tracers • Limited availability • Limited center experience

Abbreviations: CIED, cardiac implantable electronic device; CNS, central nervous system; CTA, CT angiography; NVE, native valve endocarditis; PVE, prosthetic valve endocarditis; SPECT, single-photon emission CT.

Modified from Millar BC, Habib G, Moore JE. New diagnostic approaches in infective endocarditis. Heart 2016;102:796–807.

Table 2
International guidelines relating to the use of imaging modalities to diagnose and monitor cardiac infection

Guidelines	Recommendations Relating to Imaging Modalities

Modified Duke Criteria[6]	1. Major diagnostic criteria-positive echocardiogram (TTE/TEE)
	  Echocardiogram positive for IE (TEE recommended in patients with prosthetic valves, rated at least possible IE by clinical criteria, or complicated IE [paravalvular abscess]; TTE as first test in other patients), defined as follows:
	  • Oscillating intracardiac mass on valve or supporting structures, in the path of regurgitant jets, or on implanted material in the absence of an alternative anatomic explanation, or
	  • Abscess, or
	  • New partial dehiscence of prosthetic valve
	  • New valvular regurgitation (worsening or changing of preexisting murmur not sufficient)

AHA[7]	1. Echocardiography recommendations
	  • TTE should be performed in all cases of suspected IE
	  • TEE should be done if initial TTE images are negative or inadequate in patients for whom there is an ongoing suspicion for IE or when there is concern or intracardiac complications in patients with initial positive TTE
	  • If there is a high suspicion of IE despite initial negative TEE, then repeat TEE is recommended in 3–5 d or sooner if clinical findings change
	  • Repeat TEE should be done after initially positive TEE if clinical features suggest a new development of intracardiac complications
	  • TTE at the time of antimicrobial therapy completion to establish baseline features is reasonable
	2. Other imaging modalities
	  • 3D TEE, cardiac CT, coronary CTA, PET-MRI, ^{18}F-FDG-PET/CT usage may increase in the future as the risks and benefits of each modality are defined

ESC[4]	1. Echocardiography recommendations:
	  • First-line TTE in all cases of suspected IE
	  • TEE in patients with clinical suspicion of IE and negative or nondiagnostic TTE, or in patients with clinical suspicion of IE, when a prosthetic heart valve or an intracardiac device is present
	  • When clinical suspicion of IE remains high, repeat TTE and/or TEE
	  • Cases of *Staphylococcus aureus* bacteremia
	  • If negative, repeat TTE and/or TEE during follow-up under medical therapy and for the examination of silent complications and vegetation size
	  • Intracardiac echocardiography recommended in all cases of IE requiring surgery
	  • TTE recommended following completion of therapy.
	2. In the setting of the suspicion of endocarditis on a prosthetic valve, abnormal activity around the site of implantation detected by ^{18}F-FDG-PET/CT (only if the prosthesis was implanted greater than 3 mo) or radiolabeled leukocyte SPECT/CT should be considered a major criterion
	3. The identification of paravalvular lesions by cardiac CT should be considered a major criterion
	4. The sensitivity of the Duke criteria can be improved by new imaging modalities (PET-MRI, CT, PET/CT) that allow the diagnosis of embolic events and cardiac involvement when TTE/TEE findings are negative or doubtful
	5. The identification of recent embolic events or infectious aneurysms by imaging only (silent events) should be considered a minor criterion
	6. ^{18}F-FDG-PET/CT and radiolabeled leukocyte SPECT/CT have proven roles in the diagnosis of cardiovascular electronic implanted devices, but the data are not sufficient for them to be included in the diagnostic criteria of the specific topic of IE on pacemaker or defibrillator leads

Abbreviation: 3D, three-dimensional.

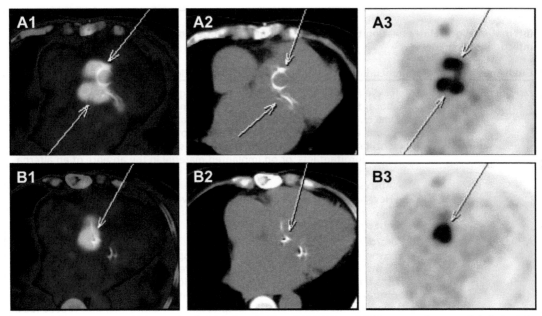

Fig. 1. Axial 18F-FDG–PET/CT (*A1* and *B1*), CT (*A2* and *B2*) and PET (*A3* and *B3*) images of a case of definite infective endocarditis (IE) in a 67-year-old patient with prosthetic aortic and mitral valves implanted 4 years previously. Histologically confirmed IE caused by Staphylococcus aureus. 18F-FDG-PET/CT showed focal areas of enhanced glycolytic metabolism around the aortic (A1 and A3 *arrows*) and mitral (B1 and B3 *arrows*) prosthetics valves, the standard uptake value was 7.6 and 6.0, respectively.

initially classified as possible to definite IE, permitting a conclusive diagnosis (definite/rejected) at admission in 97.6% of cases.[12] A separate large, 6-center study (160 patients with prosthetic valves; 62 biological, 82 mechanical, 9 transcatheter aortic valve replacement, 7 other), concluded that when[18]F-FDG-PET/CT is implemented early in the diagnostic work-up for PVE, a positive finding can occur even when conventional diagnostic parameters such as blood culture and echocardiography are negative.[13] A substantial increase in diagnostic sensitivity when ^{18}F-FDG-PET/CT was added to echocardiography findings (ie, 65% echocardiography alone to 96% with both imaging techniques combined) highlights that a positive finding on ^{18}F-FDG-PET/CT analysis can occur before any structural damage has occurred, thereby potentially permitting intervention before the occurrence of severe complications, such as perivalvular abscesses or valve dehiscence.[13]

NATIVE VALVE ENDOCARDITIS

In contrast with PVE, a review analysis of several small-scale studies[14,15] and 2 recent large retrospective studies[12,16] has suggested a low-sensitivity diagnostic value relating to ^{18}F-FDG-PET/CT when used alone, in terms of uptake of tracer in native valves in which infection has been

proved (sensitivity, specificity, positive and negative predictive values: 18%, 100%, 100%, and 66%, respectively).[12] Possible reasons for the limited sensitivity have been attributed to (1) continuous movement of cardiac valves during acquisition, (2) small size of vegetations and thus a low level of metabolism could result in difficulties in detection above background uptake and blurred image caused by heart movement, and (3) subacute phase of NVE may result in transportation of vegetations into calcium deposits and tracer normally accumulates in activated leukocytes[16] (**Fig. 2**).

However, when ^{18}F-FDG-PET/CT findings are included with the Modified Duke Criteria, an increase in positive NVE diagnoses is noted in cases originally classified as possible or rejected. Therefore, ^{18}F-FDG-PET/CT could be useful in challenging NVE cases in which there is a strong suspicion of NVE and that have been difficult to diagnose using conventional approaches.[16]

CARDIAC IMPLANTABLE ELECTRONIC DEVICE INFECTION

CIED therapy is continuing to grow, with expanding implications for use including bradycardia, tachycardia, and heart failure, resulting in 1.2 million to 1.4 million CIEDs implanted annually

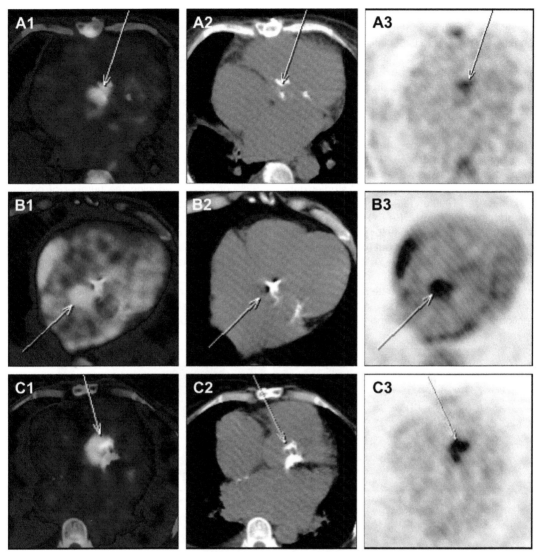

Fig. 2. Axial ^{18}F-FDG–PET/CT (A1, B1 and C1), CT (A2, B2 and C2) and PET (A3, B3 and C3) images of three distinct patients with mitral native valve endocarditis (A and B) and aortic native valve endocarditis (C). Different degrees of focal FDG uptake around the coarse calcifications in the valvar planes are shown (A1, B1, C1 and A3, B3, C3 *arrows*). The maximum standardized uptake value (SUVmax) was 2.8, 3.8 and 5.6, in A1, B1 and C1 respectively. Discrete heterogeneous ^{18}F-FDG uptake in the myocardium, predominantly in the right atrium, probably related to the metabolic demand caused by heart failure and atrial fibrillation presented, can also be observed in B1 and B3.

worldwide.[17] Associated infections are significant, not only in terms of morbidity and mortality but also with respect to health care financial implications, in terms of both hospitalization and surgical procedures. CIEDs in an increasing aging population with concomitant comorbidities, such as diabetes mellitus, heart failure, chronic obstructive pulmonary disease, and chronic kidney disease, contribute significantly as host risk factors for device-related infection.[17] The increasing prevalence of CIED infection is of concern and therefore the accurate diagnosis and corresponding treatment regimen is of utmost importance but remains a challenge, particularly when symptoms are delayed or subtle.[17]

^{18}F-FDG-PET/CT has been recognized as particularly useful when the diagnosis of pocket or lead infection cannot be confirmed by other imaging modalities, namely TEE. Of particular note, Sarrazin and colleagues[18] proposed diagnostic algorithms incorporating ^{18}F-FDG-PET/CT for the evaluation and management of patients with suspected CIED infection, namely (1) possible pocket, lead, or intravascular infection requiring complete system extraction; and (2) limited to superficial skin infection requiring antibiotic therapy. Although

such studies have shown, and continue to show, the valuable contribution that ^{18}F-FDG-PET/CT can make in relation to CIED infection, at present the ESC has not included such an approach into the European guidelines because of insufficient data.[4] This conclusion was in agreement with recent guidelines published by the British Society for Antimicrobial Chemotherapy, in conjunction with several other British cardiac societies, although the potential role that ^{18}F-FDG-PET/CT could play in selected cases in which there is a diagnostic uncertainty was acknowledged.[19] A subsequent large meta-analysis of 14 studies published between 1990 and 2017, and involving 492 patients, showed that ^{18}F-FDG-PET/CT had a high sensitivity and specificity for pocket infection, 96% and 97% respectively, but lower for lead infections or CIED-IE (sensitivity 76% and specificity 83%),[20] which concurs with other studies.[21,22]

Although most studies to date have focused on ^{18}F-FDG-PET/CT analysis, several reports have highlighted a considerable improvement in the diagnostic yield in cases of suspected IE in patients with intravascular or intracardiac prosthetic material, when using ^{18}F-FDG-PET/CT angiography (CTA), particularly in conjunction with the Modified Duke Criteria.[23–26] This imaging approach combines high sensitivity to detect infection with the high spatial resolution to define structural damage, which was highly evident in a study of adult patients with congenital heart disease and suspected IE and/or CIED infection, in which ^{18}F-FDG-PET/CTA improved diagnostic sensitivity, from 39.1% to 89%, with a conclusive diagnosis achieved in 92% of cases, reducing the number of possible CIED-IE cases (from 56% to 8%), primarily because of the reclassification of cases.[23]

Advantages of ^{18}F-FDG-PET/(CT or CTA) application in the diagnosis of CIED infection include (1) early diagnosis, thereby reducing mortality; (2) prevention of unnecessary removal of device and, as such, associated health risks and unnecessary financial implications; and (3) evaluation of extracardiac foci of infection (**Fig. 3**).

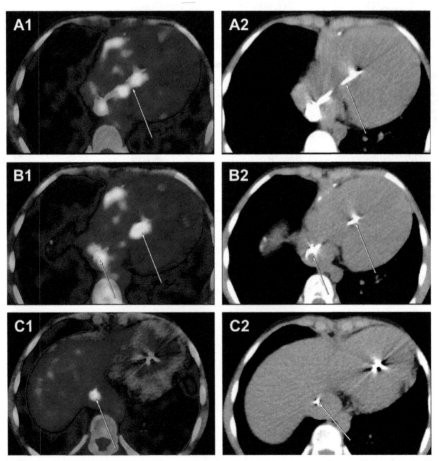

Fig. 3. Axial ^{18}F-FDG–PET/CT (*A1, B1* and *C1*) and CT (*A2, B2* and *C2*) images of a cardiac implantable electronic device (CIED) infection. 18F-FDG-PET/CT showed focal areas of enhanced glycolytic metabolism around the pacemaker lead (*A1, B1* and *C1 arrows*), the standard uptake value was 3.2.

LEFT VENTRICULAR ASSIST DEVICE INFECTION

LVADs are increasingly used to provide temporary circulatory support to patients with end-stage heart failure, both acute and chronic, that is unmanageable by medical therapy, and as such act as a bridge to transplant or destination therapy, when the patient does not meet the criteria for a transplant.[27] Other indications for use include reversible causes of heart failure (bridge to recovery) or patients who may meet the criteria for transplant in the future (bridge to candidacy).[27] LVADs have revolutionized the treatment of end-stage heart failure; however, associated complications, including infection, contribute to significant morbidity and mortality and are the most common cause of death in patients who survive the initial 6 months on LVAD support.[2] Driveline infections have been reported to be as high as 17% to 30%, and mortality following such an infection has been reported as 9.8% at 6 months and 31% at 12 months.[28] Of concern is that 20% to 40% of LVAD recipients develop sepsis within 2 years of implantation.[29] The timely diagnosis of infection is challenging but extremely important to ensure that treatment is commenced early to ensure a favorable outcome. The strongest evidence for LVAD infection is microbiological findings from swabs of the explanted driveline or device, which are generally not available. Recently the use of ^{18}F-FDG-PET/CT has shown high diagnostic capabilities in relation to driveline infection in both children[30] and adults,[31–37] which is as accurate as, and more sensitive than, leucocyte-labeled scintigraphy.[36] In contrast, the diagnostic accuracy in relation to pump housing infection is limited, and it is recommended that qualitative analyses would be better considered.[34] Possible explanations for this limitation include (1) unspecific ^{18}F-FDG uptake caused by foreign body reaction around the LVAD, (2) physiologic tracer uptake into adjacent left ventricular myocardium, (3) the presence of chronic fistula, and (4) possible infection of the inner surface of the pump housing.[34]

Although the diagnostic accuracy when using ^{18}F-FDG-PET/CT is consistently high in relation to LVAD infection regardless of the image analysis used, quantitative parameters yield a higher sensitivity and specificity than visual grading alone. A retrospective study evaluated both a qualitative and a semiquantitative approach and noted that qualitative examination of ^{18}F-FDG uptake along the driveline is seldom prone to artifacts; however, this depends on the examiner's experience and is not suitable for follow-up or interpatient and intrapatient comparison.[37] Semiquantitative analysis of ^{18}F-FDG-PET/CT can additionally improve diagnosis by comparing baseline examination using a distinctive maximum standardized uptake value (SUV_{max}) threshold of 3.88, with a sensitivity and specificity of 100% (no driveline infection, mean $\Delta SUV_{max} = 0.03 \pm 0.43$; LVAD-related infection, $\Delta SUV_{max} = 4.38 \pm 1.44$).[37] Furthermore, a comparative study of 48 patients with implanted LVADs showed that the use of metabolic volume as a metric parameter led to a further improvement in the diagnostic accuracy compared with SUV_{max}.[31]

INFECTIVE ENDOCARDITIS COMPLICATIONS

Secondary complications following IE and CIED infection are primarily associated with septic embolic events, occurring in 22% to 43% of patients, generally within the first 2 weeks of therapy, with pulmonary emboli being the most frequent.[38] Complications of IE include metastatic infection, septic arthritis, spondylodiscitis, osteomyelitis, pericarditis, and metastatic soft tissue abscess. Analyses of recent prospective and retrospective studies[38–42] have shown ^{18}F-FDG-PET/CT to be useful in detecting such complications; in many cases, ^{18}F-FDG-PET/CT is the first modality to localize such infectious metastatic foci in patients with NVE,[16] even before any clinical suggestion.[38] As such, the ESC guidelines recommend ^{18}F-FDG-PET/CT to be used in conjunction with other imaging investigations, such as cerebral PET-MRI and whole-body CT, to aid in the investigation of embolic events[4] (**Figs. 4** and **5**).

GRAFT INFECTION

Prosthetic graft infections can be associated with prosthetic valves, aortic vascular stent prostheses, or hybrid prostheses. Early superficial wound infection occurs in 3.2% of cases and endocarditis occurs as a late complication in 1.4% of cases.[43] Such infections are potentially life threatening and treatment may involve repeat surgery, which is associated with a high morbidity and mortality; however, currently there are no specific diagnostic criteria available to ensure the optimum diagnosis for graft infections. Diagnosis of valved aortic graft infection has predominantly relied on TTE, TEE, and CT imaging; however, more recently several groups have documented the potential role that ^{18}F-FDG-PET/CT could play in the assessment of suspected aortic grafts/valved aortic graft infection.[3,44–46]

A recent case series and systematic review of the literature examining such graft infections acknowledged that, if TEE and CT findings are negative,

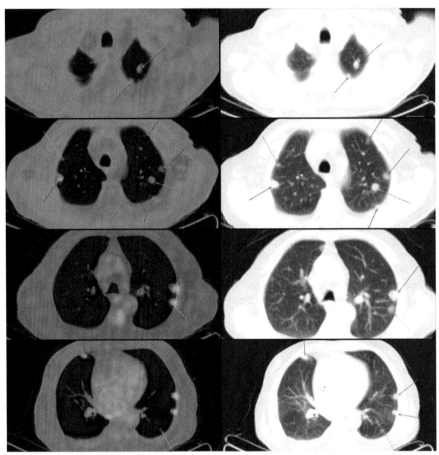

Fig. 4. Axial ^{18}F-FDG-PET/CT and CT images of a patient with definite NVE with extensive lung septic emboli.

^{18}F-FDG-PET/CT or SPEC/CT can potentially play key roles in the diagnosis of Bentall graft infections.[3] This finding echoed previous advice that CT and echocardiography, if applicable, should remain the first diagnostic steps in cases of suspected graft infections following cardiac surgery, primarily because of availability and because false-positive results caused by ^{18}F-FDG accumulation may occur because of chronic inflammatory reactions or postoperative changes, particularly within the first 8 -week postoperative period. ^{18}F-FDG-PET/CT should be reserved subsequently, either for confirmation or when diagnosis is not achievable by conventional methods[46] **(Fig. 6).**

MONITORING OF ANTIMICROBIAL THERAPY

It is recognized that the duration of antimicrobial therapy in the treatment of IE infection varies depending on the site of infection (NVE, PVE, or CIED infection) and the causative organism. Treatment durations are based either on randomized studies conducted in the 1990s or on expert opinion, with a lack of recent comparative

data on treatment duration with respect to IE.[47] The promising role of ^{18}F-FDG-PET/CT in the monitoring of antimicrobial therapy in IE has been suggested by small observational studies that have provided evidence both for resolution of infection following long-term antimicrobial therapy[48] and the persistence of infection at the end of standard treatment, thus determining a need for continued therapy until the normalization of metabolic activity was achieved.[49] Further large-scale studies are therefore warranted to further investigate this application **(Fig. 7).**

OTHER CARDIAC INFECTIONS

There have been several interesting case reports in which ^{18}F-FDG-PET has been reported to be beneficial in the detection other cardiac-related infections and unusual localizations of IE, such as endarteritis of the descending aorta,[50] myocardial tuberculoma,[51] mural endocarditis,[52] myocarditis,[53,54] infected left ventricular pseudoaneurysm,[55] and infected pulmonary conduit.[56,57]

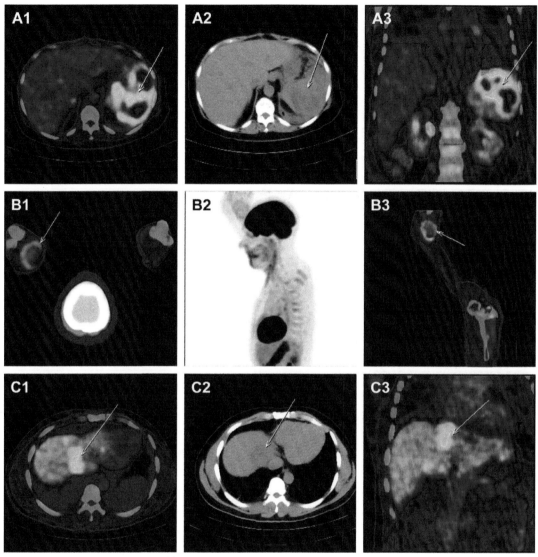

Fig. 5. Axial, sagittal and coronal ^{18}F-FDG–PET/CT images of three patients with infective endocarditis and systemic emboli. (A1 and A3 *arrows*). Extensive splenic emboli, (B1 and B3 *arrows*) mycotic pseudoaneurysm and (C1 and C3 *arrows*) liver emboli.

LIMITATIONS AND SUGGESTED IMPROVEMENTS

A major limitation to the application ^{18}F-FDG-PET/CT in the diagnosis of cardiac infection is the current lack of standardized protocols in relation to both patient preparation and image interpretation, which may have contributed to the variation of findings in the published literature. A recent extensive analysis of current protocols has been conducted in an attempt to construct an evidence-based practice in order to improve the diagnostic potential of ^{18}F-FDG-PET/CT in relation to PVE and CIED infection.[58]

Of primary concern is the difficulty associated with the physiologic uptake of tracer by the normal myocardium, which may mask the pathologic uptake[59] (**Fig. 8**). Patient preparation methods have therefore been proposed, before tracer administration, to inhibit or block such normal physiologic uptake, which is possible because there are independent mechanisms of glucose incorporation in cardiomyocytes, namely the glucose transporter type 4 (GLUT-4), whereas in inflammatory cells this is mediated via GLUT-1 and GLUT-3 transporters.[58]

Specific diet models, low in carbohydrate, rich in fat and proteins, suitable for both diabetic and nondiabetic patients, have been proposed for a

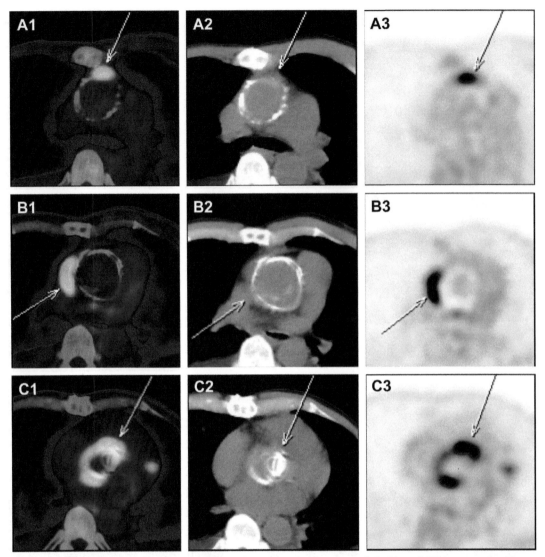

Fig. 6. Axial ^{18}F-FDG–PET/CT (A1, B1 and C1), CT (A2, B2 and C2) and PET (A3, B3 and C3) images of a 62-year-old patient with Bentall De Bono prosthesis (ascending aortic prosthesis plus prosthetic aortic valve) implanted 10 years previously and definite infective endocarditis (IE) resulting from coagulase-negative staphylococci. The PET/CT showed intense focal uptake around the ascending aortic tube (A1, A3, B1 and B3 *arrows*), and in the aortic prosthetic valve (C1 and C3 *arrows*). The maximum standardized uptake value (SUVmax) was 7.6 and 7.8, respectively.

period of 24 to 72 hours.[58] In addition, many studies have implemented a 12-hour fasting period, to reduce circulating glucose and insulin levels; however, the most effective results have been achieved with a fasting period of 18 hours, when glycemia levels are at their lowest and circulating fatty acid levels are at their highest.[58,59] Furthermore, a bolus of unfractionated heparin (50 IU/kg, 1%, 10–15 minutes before tracer) not only blocks myocardial blockade but stimulates lipolytic activity by activating lipoproteins and hepatic and blood lipases, thereby increasing fatty acid concentrations in blood, which may be used as first energy sources by myocardial cells.[58,60] Because increased blood glucose competes with ^{18}FDG for uptake at sites of infection, deferring ^{18}F-FDG-PET/CT is recommend if the patient's blood sugar level is greater than 200 mg/dL. Although most studies have adopted acquisition times typically a 1-hour period, following ^{18}FDG injection, it has been reported that a better target-to-background ratio is achievable if imaging is delayed to 90 minutes, with one report noting a further improvement at later acquisition times of 2 to 3 hours.[61]

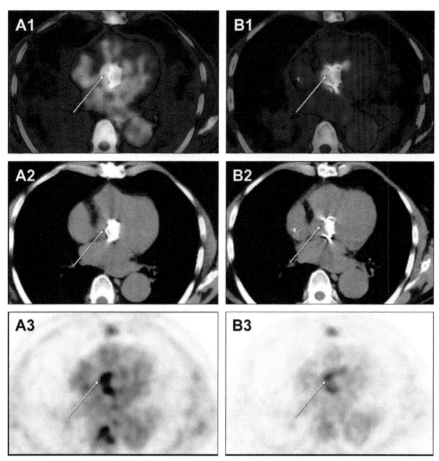

Fig. 7. Axial ^{18}F-FDG–PET/CT (A1 and B1), CT (A2 and B2) and PET (A3 and B3) images of two consecutive scans of the same patient with an aortic prosthetic valve, (A1 and A3 *arrows*) The PET/CT showed intense focal uptake around the aortic prosthetic valve (SUVmax: 5.4), in a patient with definite infective endocarditis (IE) caused by viridans streptococci, (B1 *arrow*). Follow-up PET/CT after 6 weeks (42 days with antibiotic therapy) showed decrease of tracer uptake around the valvar planes (SUVmax: 3.3), associated with a change in the uptake pattern which became diffuse (B3 *arrow*).

FALSE FINDINGS

False-negative findings have been attributed to low inflammatory activity at the time of imaging, possibly caused by prolonged antibiotic therapy.[13] On assessment of inflammatory activity and ^{18}F-FDG-PET/CT in the diagnosis of PVE, it was reported that a C-reactive protein level of less than 4 times the upper normal limit (<40 mg/L) was a significant and major predictor of false-negative interpretations.[13] False-positive findings in areas where surgical adhesives had been applied have been noted, which may persist for extensive periods of time (years or even indefinitely)[13,59] **(Fig. 9)**. Although it has been suggested that ^{18}F-FDG-PET/CT is unreliable during the early 2- month postoperative period[11] and the ESC have stated that ^{18}F-FDG-PET/CT should only be used if the prosthesis has been implanted for 3 months,[4] Swart and colleagues[13] concluded from their study and analysis

of numerous previous studies that this was not a significant predictor of false-positive findings and, as such, poses no significant diagnostic difficulties.

IMAGE INTERPRETATION

Most studies to date have focused on visual interpretation of images, to differentiate between normal physiologic and pathologic uptake. Such visual assessment of ^{18}F-FDG-PET/CT has been reported as having a sensitivity, specificity, positive predictive value, and negative predictive value for PVE of 74%, 91%, 89%, and 78%, respectively, although this was significantly improved when patients were excluded because of significant confounders, as outlined earlier (91%, 95%, 95%, and 91%).[13]

A semiquantitative measurement of the metabolic activity of a lesion with the aid of the SUV would be less subjective and offer a more

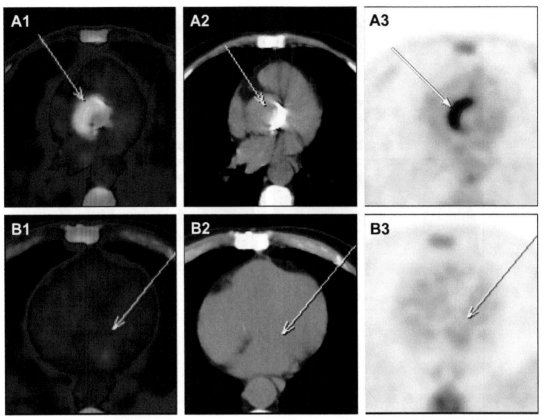

Fig. 8. Axial ^{18}F-FDG–PET/CT (A1 and B1), CT (A2 and B2) and PET (A3 and B3) images of a 68-year-old patient with histologically confirmed bivalvar endocarditis (A-prosthetic aortic valve and B-native mitral valve), caused by viridans streptococci. ^{18}F-FDG-PET/CT images showed (A1 *arrow*) intense focal uptake around the prosthetic aortic valve (SUVmax: 5.8) and (B2 *arrow*) physiological uptake around the native mitral valve (false negative).

objective cutoff value to determine pathologic significance. To help achieve this goal, published SUV values for PVE have been analyzed; however, it was concluded that they were not interchangeable between centers and varied substantially across studies, primarily because of differences in unstandardized protocols, with SUV values ranging in terms of median SUV_{max} for rejected PVE (0.5–4.9) and for definite PVE (4.2–7.4).[62] More recently, a semiquantitative measure of ^{18}F-FDG uptake, specifically an The European Association of Nuclear Medicine (EANM) Research Ltd (EARL)-standardized SUV ratio of greater than or equal to 2.0, was a 100% sensitive and 91% specific predictor of PVE.[13] It has been further suggested that the precise quantification of valvular ^{18}F-FDG uptake as intense, moderate, mild, or absent would be more appropriate than positive or negative and, as such, a registry could be established to correlate each level of uptake with probability of PVE in patients, similar to echocardiography in the Modified Duke Criteria.[63]

In relation to PVE and CIED device infection, in the absence of a clear SUV_{max} threshold for the presence of IE, both systematic use of the attenuation correction (AC) PET images and PET images with no AC (NAC) has been advocated in a qualitative and semiquantitative analysis.[21] Although NAC PET images are difficult to evaluate quantitatively, because they usually present a very low spatial resolution, especially in small lesions, they are important when evaluating cardiac infection in the presence of metallic components.[21] It has been suggested that only in cases in which areas have a lower comparative uptake of less than twice that of the liver is it necessary to evaluate the NAC PET images to minimize the likelihood of a false-positive.[21] In addition, metal artifact reduction algorithms may improve the reliability of AC image interpretation in patients with such metallic cardiac devices and valves in which artifacts such as beam hardening and scatter may occur and affect the CT-based AC and in turn the resulting AC PET images.[64]

Although within the last 3 years, larger-scale studies have been conducted in relation to IE and associated cardiac infections, there is an

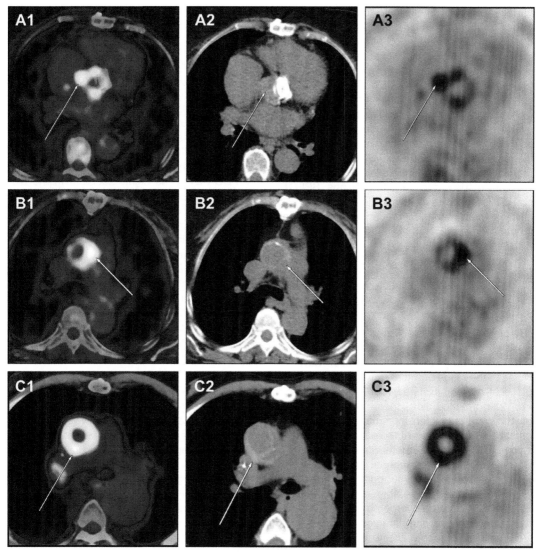

Fig. 9. Axial ^{18}F-FDG–PET/CT (A1, B1 and C1), CT (A2, B2 and C2) and PET (A3, B3 and C3) images of two distinct patients with Bentall De Bono prosthesis (ascending aortic prosthesis plus prosthetic aortic valve), without prosthetic valve endocarditis. (A and B) 63-year-old patient with Bentall De Bono prosthesis implanted 6 years previously. The PET/CT showed intense focal uptake around the aortic prosthetic valve (A1 and A3 *arrows*) and ascending aortic tube (B1 and B3 *arrows*). The maximum standardized uptake value (SUVmax) was 5.4 and 6.9, respectively. The histologically analysis excluded IE, and showed giant cell reaction related to a suture and surgical adhesive. (C) 60-year-old patient with Bentall De Bono prosthesis implanted 8 years previously. The PET/CT showed intense diffuse uptake around the ascending aortic tube with a focal uptake area (C1 and C3 *arrows*), the standard uptake value was 6.9. The two cases were considered false positives.

urgent requirement for a consensus guideline to address patient preparation, ^{18}F-FDG dosage, uptake period, acquisition period, and processing image protocols, including the inclusion of motion correction methods such as cardiac and respiratory gating and interpretation of images, subsequently enabling multicenter studies to further evaluate the role of ^{18}F-FDG-PET in the diagnosis and monitoring of cardiac infection.

LIMITATIONS AND CHALLENGES RELATED TO IMAGING THE INFECTED HEART

Over the past 5 decades, significant advances have been made in assessing structural and functional abnormalities that are associated with various diseases and disorders.[65–73] In particular, the introduction of CT and PET-MRI has substantially improved the ability to visualize anatomic structures with great detail in health and disease.

Although early instruments had the disadvantage of low spatial resolution and required image acquisition over a long period of time, modern instruments have substantially overcome these deficiencies. Similarly, the quality of functional images acquired with SPECT and PET has significantly improved with the introduction of sophisticated machines. In general, SPECT and PET scans have lower spatial resolution compared with CT and require data collection over an extended time. As such, constant physiologic motion during data acquisition further degrades image quality. However, in spite of these shortcomings, SPECT and PET are highly sensitive in detecting disease activity in many settings. In recent years, with the introduction of PET-CT, SPECT-CT, and PET-MRI, clinicians are able to determine changes that occur in both structural and functional domains in a single session. It must be emphasized that, overall, PET is superior to SPECT in providing higher image quality and covering extensive functional domains.

By now, it is well established that in order to visualize sites of abnormal uptake by PET or SPECT, the targeted structures must have a volume in the range of 5 to 8 mm^3 with significant uptake of the administered radiotracer.[74] Therefore, performance of these modalities in detecting and characterizing small lesions is suboptimal. Furthermore, as noted earlier, spatial resolution of SPECT or PET deteriorates significantly with physiologic motion (cardiac and respiratory movements) and results in suboptimal image quality. However, the undesirable effects of these movements cannot be overcome substantially by physiologic gating during data acquisition.[75]

Attempts have been made to directly visualize bacteria in various locations in the body by synthesizing specific radiotracers that target bacteria.[76] These approaches have been of limited value because of the biological nature of bacterial infections and the volume of the affected site. It is unlikely that a large volume of bacteria can accumulate at One site and reach a substantial volume without being phagocytized by the white cells. Therefore, compounds that are designed to target bacteria may never reach these organisms and allow imaging of the infected sites.

Overall, challenges that clinicians face in detecting and characterizing disease sites in the infected heart with either structural or functional imaging techniques are significant and will require further improvement in imaging techniques. Until and unless these physical and biological obstacles are overcome, the performance of modern imaging will be limited in this serious and potentially fatal infection.

SUMMARY

The role of ^{18}F-FDG-PET/CT in the diagnostic algorithm for cardiac infections should be acknowledged, particularly when used in conjunction with the Modified Duke Criteria in relation to PVE, because it is a useful adjuvant in classifying cases. ^{18}F-FDG-PET/CT should be restricted to cases of NVE with a strong suspicion of IE, but inconclusive by conventional approaches, because inclusion with the Modified Duke Criteria improves specificity in such cases. In relation to LVAD, ^{18}F-FDG-PET/CT is highly accurate in the diagnosis of driveline infection but more limited in pump housing infection. ^{18}F-FDG-PET/CT has potential in aiding in decisions concerning treatment regimens relating to CIED infection, as well as the monitoring of antimicrobial therapy in cases of IE. In all cases of IE, whole-body ^{18}F-FDG-PET/CT is beneficial in the early detection of metastatic infection and embolic events. The benefits of using ^{18}F-FDG-PET/CT in relation to cardiac infection will be further elucidated with the development of universal standardized protocols and large-scale prospective studies.

REFERENCES

1. Murillo H, Restrepo CS, Marmol-Velez JA, et al. Infectious diseases of the heart: pathophysiology, clinical and imaging overview. Radiographics 2016;36: 963–83.
2. Trachtenberg BH, Cordero-Reyes A, Elias B, et al. A review of infections in patients with left ventricular assist devices: prevention, diagnosis and management. Methodist Debakey Cardiovasc J 2015;11: 28–32.
3. Machelart I, Greib C, Wirth G, et al. Graft infection after a Bentall procedure: a case series and systematic review of the literature. Diagn Microbiol Infect Dis 2017;88:158–62.
4. Habib G, Lancellotti P, Antunes MJ, et al. 2015 ESC guidelines for the management of infective endocarditis: The Task Force for the Management of Infective Endocarditis of the European Society of Cardiology (ESC). Endorsed by: European Association for Cardio-Thoracic Surgery (EACTS), the European Association of Nuclear Medicine (EANM). Eur Heart J 2015;36:3075–128.
5. Millar BC, Habib G, Moore JE. New diagnostic approaches in infective endocarditis. Heart 2016;102: 796–807.
6. Li JS, Sexton DJ, Mick N, et al. Proposed modifications to the Duke criteria for the diagnosis of infective endocarditis. Clin Infect Dis 2000;30:633–8.
7. Baddour LM, Wilson WR, Bayer AS, et al. Infective endocarditis in adults: diagnosis, antimicrobial

therapy, and management of complications: a scientific statement for healthcare professionals from the American Heart Association. Circulation 2015;132:1435–86.

8. Millar B, Moore J, Mallon P, et al. Molecular diagnosis of infective endocarditis–a new Duke's criterion. Scand J Infect Dis 2001;33:673–80.

9. Tak T, Shukla SK. Molecular diagnosis of infective endocarditis: a helpful addition to the Duke criteria. Clin Med Res 2004;2:206–8.

10. Faraji R, Behjati-Ardakani M, Faraji N, et al. Molecular diagnosis of bacterial definite infective endocarditis by real-time polymerase chain reaction. Cardiol Res 2018;9:99–106.

11. Balmforth D, Chacko J, Uppal R. Does positron emission tomography/computed tomography aid the diagnosis of prosthetic valve infective endocarditis? Interact Cardiovasc Thorac Surg 2016;23:648–52.

12. Camargo RA, Siciliano RF, Paixao MR, et al. Diagnostic value of positron emission tomography (PET/CT) in native and prosthetic infective endocarditis. Eur Heart J 2017;38(Issue Suppl 1):1010.

13. Swart LE, Gomes A, Scholtens AM, et al. Improving the diagnostic performance of ^{18}F-FDG PET/CT in prosthetic heart valve endocarditis. Circulation 2018;138:1412–27.

14. Millar BC, Prendergast BD, Alavi A, et al. [18]FDG-positron emission tomography (PET) has a role to play in the diagnosis and therapy of infective endocarditis and cardiac device infection. Int J Cardiol 2013;167:1724–36.

15. Gomes A, Glaudemans AWJM, Touw DJ, et al. Diagnostic value of imaging in infective endocarditis: a systematic review. Lancet Infect Dis 2017;17:e1–14.

16. Kouijzer IJE, Berrevoets MAH, Aarntzen EHJG, et al. ^{18}F-fluorodeoxyglucose positron-emission tomography combined with computed tomography as a diagnostic tool in native valve endocarditis. Nucl Med Commun 2018;39:747–52.

17. Kusumoto FM, Schoenfeld MH, Wilkoff BL. 2017 HRS expert consensus statement on cardiovascular implantable electronic device lead management and extraction. Heart Rhythm 2017;14:e503–51.

18. Sarrazin JF, Philippon F, Tessier M, et al. Usefulness of fluorine-18 positron emission tomography/computed tomography for identification of cardiovascular implantable electronic device infections. J Am Coll Cardiol 2012;59:1616–25.

19. Sandoe JA, Barlow G, Chambers JB, et al. New guidelines for prevention and management of implantable cardiac electronic device-related infection. Lancet 2015;38:2225–6.

20. Mahmood M, Kendi AT, Farid S, et al. Role of ^{18}F-FDG PET/CT in the diagnosis of cardiovascular implantable electronic device infections: a meta-

analysis. J Nucl Cardiol 2017. https://doi.org/10.1007/s12350-017-1063-0.

21. Jiménez-Ballvé A, Pérez-Castejón MJ, Delgado-Bolton RC, et al. Assessment of the diagnostic accuracy of 18F-FDG PET/CT in prosthetic infective endocarditis and cardiac implantable electronic device infection: comparison of different interpretation criteria. Eur J Nucl Med Mol Imaging 2016;43:2401–12.

22. Juneau D, Golfam M, Hazra S, et al. Positron emission tomography and single-photon emission computed tomography imaging in the diagnosis of cardiac implantable electronic device infection: a systematic review and meta-analysis. Circ Cardiovasc Imaging 2017;10 [pii:e005772].

23. Pizzi MN, Dos-Subirà L, Roque A, et al. ^{18}F-FDG-PET/CT angiography in the diagnosis of infective endocarditis and cardiac device infection in adult patients with congenital heart disease and prosthetic material. Int J Cardiol 2017;248:396–402.

24. Aguadé-Bruix S, Pizzi MN, Roque A, et al. Diagnostic value of 18F-FDG PET/cardiac CT in late prosthetic aortic endocarditis with periprosthetic abscess. Rev Esp Med Nucl Imagen Mol 2017;36(1):59–60.

25. Lozano-Torres J, Pizzi MN, Roque A, et al. Recurrent prosthetic mitral valve infective endocarditis and perivalvular abscess: first description by PET/CT angiography. Eur J Nucl Med Mol Imaging 2016;43:1565.

26. Roque A, Pizzi MN, Cuéllar-Calàbria H, et al. ^{18}F-FDG-PET/CT angiography for the diagnosis of infective endocarditis. Curr Cardiol Rep 2017;19:15.

27. Kadakia S, Moore R, Ambur V, et al. Current status of the implantable LVAD. Gen Thorac Cardiovasc Surg 2016;64:501–8.

28. Koval CE, Thuita L, Moazami N, et al. Evolution and impact of drive-line infection in a large cohort of continuous-flow ventricular assist device recipients. J Heart Lung Transplant 2014;33:1164–72.

29. Legallois D, Manrique A. Diagnosis of infection in patients with left ventricular assist device: PET or SPECT? J Nucl Cardiol 2018. https://doi.org/10.1007/s12350-018-1324-6.

30. Absi M, Bocchini C, Price JF, et al. F-fluorodeoxyglucose-positive emission tomography/CT imaging for left ventricular assist device-associated infections in children. Cardiol Young 2018;28:1157–9.

31. Avramovic N, Dell'Aquila AM, Weckesser M, et al. Metabolic volume performs better than SUVmax in the detection of left ventricular assist device drive-line infection. Eur J Nucl Med Mol Imaging 2017;44:1870–7.

32. Bernhardt AM, Pamirsad MA, Brand C, et al. The value of fluorine-18 deoxyglucose positron emission tomography scans in patients with ventricular assist

device specific infections. Eur J Cardiothorac Surg 2017;51:1072–7.

33. Akin S, Muslem R, Constantinescu AA, et al. ^{18}F-FDG PET/CT in the diagnosis and management of continuous flow left ventricular assist device infections: a case series and review of the literature. ASAIO J 2018;64:e11–9.

34. Dell'Aquila AM, Avramovic N, Mastrobuoni S, et al. Fluorine-18 fluorodeoxyglucose positron emission tomography/computed tomography for improving diagnosis of infection in patients on CF-LVAD: longing for more 'insights'. Eur Heart J Cardiovasc Imaging 2018;19:532–43.

35. Kim J, Feller ED, Chen W, et al. FDG PET/CT for early detection and localization of left ventricular assist device infection: impact on patient management and outcome. JACC Cardiovasc Imaging 2018. https://doi.org/10.1016/j.jcmg.2018.01.024.

36. de Vaugelade C, Mesguich C, Nubret K, et al. Infections in patients using ventricular-assist devices: comparison of the diagnostic performance of ^{18}F-FDG PET/CT scan and leucocyte-labeled scintigraphy. J Nucl Cardiol 2018. https://doi.org/10.1007/s12350-018-1323-7.

37. Kanapinn P, Burchert W, Körperich H, et al. ^{18}F-FDG PET/CT-imaging of left ventricular assist device infection: a retrospective quantitative intrapatient analysis. J Nucl Cardiol 2018. https://doi.org/10.1007/s12350-017-1161-z.

38. Van Riet J, Hill EE, Gheysens O, et al. (18)F-FDG PET/CT for early detection of embolism and metastatic infection in patients with infective endocarditis. Eur J Nucl Med Mol Imaging 2010; 37:1189–97.

39. Orvin K, Goldberg E, Bernstine H, et al. The role of FDG-PET/CT imaging in early detection of extracardiac complications of infective endocarditis. Clin Microbiol Infect 2015;21:69–76.

40. Amraoui S, Tlili G, Sohal M, et al. Contribution of PET imaging to the diagnosis of septic embolism in patients with pacing lead endocarditis. JACC Cardiovasc Imaging 2016;9:283–90.

41. Granados U, Fuster D, Pericas JM, et al. Diagnostic accuracy of ^{18}F-FDG PET/CT in infective endocarditis and implantable cardiac electronic device infection: a cross-sectional study. J Nucl Med 2016;57: 1726–32.

42. Mikail N, Benali K, Mahida B, et al. ^{18}F-FDG-PET/CT Imaging to diagnose septic emboli and mycotic aneurysms in patients with endocarditis and cardiac device infections. Curr Cardiol Rep 2018;20:14.

43. Joo HC, Chang BC, Youn YN, et al. Clinical experience with the Bentall procedure: 28 years. Yonsei Med J 2012;53:915–23.

44. García-Arribas D, Vilacosta I, Ortega Candil A, et al. Usefulness of positron emission tomography/

computed tomography in patients with valve-tube graft infection. Heart 2018;104:1447–54.

45. Mikail N, Benali K, Dossier A, et al. Additional diagnostic value of combined angio-computed tomography and ^{18}F-fluorodeoxyglucose positron emission tomography in infectious aortitis. JACC Cardiovasc Imaging 2018;11(2 Pt 2):361–4.

46. Guenther SPW, Cyran CC, Rominger A, et al. The relevance of 18F-fluorodeoxyglucose positron emission tomography/computed tomography imaging in diagnosing prosthetic graft infections post cardiac and proximal thoracic aortic surgery. Interact Cardiovasc Thorac Surg 2015;21:450–8.

47. Wintenberger C, Guery B, Bonnet E, et al. Proposal for shorter antibiotic therapies. Med Mal Infect 2017; 47:92–141.

48. Puerta-Alcalde P, Cuervo G, Simonetti AF, et al. PET/CT added to Duke criteria facilitates diagnosis and monitoring of long-term suppressive therapy of prosthetic endocarditis. Infect Dis (Lond) 2017;49: 698–701.

49. García JR, Fortuny C, Riaza L, et al. Diagnosis by (18)F-FDG PET/CT of infective endocarditis, staging and monitoring of antibiotic treatment after transposition of surgically corrected great arteries. Rev Esp Med Nucl Imagen Mol 2016;35:115–7.

50. Sinan ÜY, Dirlik Serim B, Yıldırım R, et al. Endarteritis of coarctation of the aorta diagnosed with PET-CT. Turk Kardiyol Dern Ars 2018;46:66–8.

51. Braquet P, Baptista G, Ilonca DA, et al. FDG-PET in a myocardial tuberculoma. Age Ageing 2015;44: 173–4.

52. Litmathe J, Fussen R, Heinzel A, et al. An unusual agent for an unusual localization of infective endocarditis. Perfusion 2017;32:691–4.

53. von Olshausen G, Hyafil F, Langwieser N, et al. Detection of acute inflammatory myocarditis in Epstein Barr virus infection using hybrid ^{18}F-fluoro-deoxyglucose-positron emission tomography/magnetic resonance imaging. Circulation 2014;130:925–6.

54. Sperry BW, Oldan JD, Hsich EM, et al. Infectious myocarditis on FDG-PET imaging mimicking sarcoidosis. J Nucl Cardiol 2015;22:840–4.

55. Roosens B, Argacha JF, Soens L, et al. Left ventricular pseudo-aneurysm as a source of recurrent septicaemia. Eur Heart J Cardiovasc Imaging 2017;18:94.

56. Zhang Y, Williams H, Pucar D. FDG-PET identification of infected pulmonary artery conduit following tetralogy of Fallot (TOF) repair. Nucl Med Mol Imaging 2017;51:86–7.

57. Bonou M, Kapelios CJ, Samarkos M, et al. Early diagnosis of right ventricle-pulmonary artery conduit endocarditis by PET/CT. Int J Infect Dis 2018;68: 24–5.

58. Aguadé Bruix S, Roque Pérez A, Cuéllar Calabria H, et al. Cardiac 18F-FDG PET/CT procedure for the diagnosis of prosthetic endocarditis and

intracardiac devices. Rev Esp Med Nucl Imagen Mol 2018;37:163–71.

59. Scholtens AM, Swart LE, Verberne HJ, et al. Confounders in FDG-PET/CT imaging of suspected prosthetic valve endocarditis. JACC Cardiovasc Imaging 2016;9:1462–5.

60. Scholtens AM, Verberne HJ, Budde RP, et al. Additional heparin preadministration improves cardiac glucose metabolism suppression over low-carbohydrate diet alone in ^{18}F-FDG PET imaging. J Nucl Med 2016;57:568–73.

61. Caldarella C, Leccisotti L, Treglia G, et al. Which is the optimal acquisition time for FDG PET/CT imaging in patients with infective endocarditis? J Nucl Cardiol 2013;20:307–9.

62. Scholtens AM, Swart LE, Kolste HJT, et al. Standardized uptake values in FDG PET/CT for prosthetic heart valve endocarditis: a call for standardization. J Nucl Cardiol 2018;25:2084–91.

63. Hyafil F, Rouzet F, Le Guludec D. Quantification of FDG uptake in patients with a suspicion of prosthetic valve endocarditis: part of the problem or part of the solution? J Nucl Cardiol 2018;25:2092–5.

64. Scholtens AM, Verberne HJ. Attenuation correction and metal artifact reduction in FDG PET/CT for prosthetic heart valve and cardiac implantable device endocarditis. J Nucl Cardiol 2018;25:2172–3.

65. Alavi A, Reivich M. Guest editorial: the conception of FDG-PET imaging. Semin Nucl Med 2002;32:2–5.

66. Anger HO. Scintillation camera. Rev Sci Instrum 1958;29:27–33.

67. Hounsfield GN. Computerized transverse axial scanning (tomography). 1. description of system. Br J Radiol 1973;46:1016–22.

68. Keyes JW Jr, Orlandea N, Heetderks WJ, et al. The Humongotron–a scintillation-camera transaxial tomograph. J Nucl Med 1977;18:381–7.

69. Kuhl DE, Edwards RQ. Image separation radioisotope scanning. Radiology 1963;80:653–62.

70. Kuhl DE, Edwards RQ, Ricci AR, et al. The Mark IV system for radionuclide computed tomography of the brain. Radiology 1976;121:405–13.

71. Kuhl DE, Reivich M, Alavi A, et al. Local cerebral blood volume determined by three-dimensional reconstruction of radionuclide scan data. Circ Res 1975;36:610–9.

72. Lauterbur PC. Image formation by induced local interactions: examples employing nuclear magnetic resonance. Nature 1973;242:190–1.

73. Ter-Pogossian MM, Phelps ME, Hoffman EJ, et al. A positron-emission transaxial tomograph for nuclear imaging (PETT). Radiology 1975;114:89–98.

74. Alavi A, Werner TJ, Høilund-Carlsen PF. What can be and what cannot be accomplished with PET: rectifying ongoing misconceptions. Clin Nucl Med 2017;42:603–5.

75. Salavati A, Borofsky S, Boon-Keng TK, et al. Application of partial volume effect correction and 4D PET in the quantification of FDG avid lung lesions. Mol Imaging Biol 2015;17:140–8.

76. Hess S, Alavi A, Werner T, et al. Molecular imaging of bacteria in patients is an attractive fata morgana, not a realistic option. J Nucl Med 2018;59:716–7.

Gating Approaches in Cardiac PET Imaging

Martin Lyngby Lassen, PhD[a,1], Jacek Kwiecinski, MD[a,b,1], Piotr J. Slomka, PhD[a,*]

KEYWORDS

• Cardiac imaging • Respiratory gating • Cardiac gating • PET/CT imaging • PET/MR imaging

KEY POINTS

- Cardiac and respiratory motion has a detrimental effect on cardiovascular PET imaging and affects both quantitative and qualitative PET measures.
- Gating can ameliorate the unfavorable impact of motion additionally enabling evaluation of left ventricular systolic function (ejection fraction) and wall motion abnormalities.
- Cardiac gating is used in the clinical setting, whereas respiratory motion gating remains a research tool.

INTRODUCTION

PET is a powerful, quantitative imaging modality that has been used for decades to non-invasively investigate cardiovascular biology and physiology.[1] The PET images are, however, affected by physiologic patient motion, which degrades the images qualitatively as well as quantitatively. Three distinct motion patterns can be observed in thoracic PET scans: cardiac contraction, respiratory motion, and patient repositioning during the acquisition. In this review, the authors discuss recent advances in cardiac and respiratory gating and provide an overview of the most promising recent developments in the field.

CLINICAL BACKGROUND

Because of its superior sensitivity, spatial and temporal resolution compared with single-photon emission computed tomography, PET has been considered the gold standard for noninvasive

assessment of myocardial perfusion and viability.[2,3] Its potential extends beyond the assessment of coronary artery disease (CAD) patients. PET facilitates early diagnosis of a broad range of cardiac conditions, which affect the myocardium, such as cardiomyopathies,[4,5] infiltrative myocardial disease including sarcoidosis,[6,7] and amyloidosis.[8] Furthermore, PET plays a key role in the detection of endocarditis[9] and inflammation related to implantable device infection.[10] Recently, cardiac PET imaging is also undergoing clinical validation in the assessment of unstable coronary plaques, which are at high risk of rupture.[11–14]

MODERN PET SYSTEMS

Aside from the development of novel tracers, the improvement in the clinical assessment of cardiac disease has partly been facilitated through the continuous improvement in the spatial resolution of the PET systems, which in current PET/computed tomographic (CT) systems reaches 2

Disclosure: This work was supported in part by grant (R01HL135557) from the National Heart, Lung, and Blood Institute/National Institute of Health (NHLBI/NIH). The content is solely the responsibility of the authors and does not necessarily represent the official views of the National Institutes of Health.
[a] Cedars-Sinai Medical Center, 8700 Beverly Boulevard, Los Angeles, CA 90048, USA; [b] British Heart Foundation Centre for Cardiovascular Science, University of Edinburgh, Edinburgh, UK
[1] These authors contributed equally to the article.
* Corresponding author. 8700 Beverly Boulevard, Suite A047N, Los Angeles, CA 90048.
E-mail address: Piotr.Slomka@cshs.org

to 5 mm at full-width at half maximum.[15,16] Correction for point spread function as well as time-of-flight imaging has become standard in many modern PET systems, which offer improved localization of the annihilation event and thus improved spatial recovery of the tracer distribution.[17–20] The high-resolution PET systems, in theory, permit accurate delineation of abnormal areas with a precision similar to the PET scanner's spatial resolution.[11,12,21–23] Unfortunately, high-resolution imaging of the myocardium is hampered by motion during the acquisitions.[24] The detrimental impact of motion during the PET acquisition was recognized already in 1982 when it was proposed to divide the PET data into motion-limited bins based on the respiratory/cardiac phase.[25]

Since then, several studies have investigated the effects of cardiac and respiratory motion.[26–30] The most investigated has been the correction for the cardiac contraction, despite the fact that other motion patterns have equally detrimental effects on image quality.[31,32] One reason for this is the potential need for additional equipment to track the respiratory motion patterns.

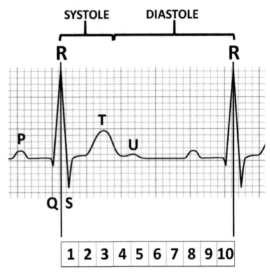

Fig. 1. Principle of ECG-gating shown using an 10-bin ECG-gating. The acquired PET data for each R-R interval is divided into a user-specified number of phases of the cardiac contraction.

CARDIAC GATING

Nowadays, in the clinical setting usually 3-lead electrocardiogram (ECG) is used.[33] With the lead data being directly transferred to the scanner, both retrospective and prospective gating of the acquired PET is feasible. The use of 3-lead ECG is relatively easy and cheap and has been shown to be reproducible in many studies.[34] Aside from the gating functionality, it also serves to monitor the patient during the acquisition. The acquired ECG signal uses the R wave as a reference to estimate the cardiac phase in which each coincidence was acquired, ultimately allowing the data to be sorted into near motion-free cardiac gates (**Fig. 1**). Cardiac gating in most modern systems is performed retrospectively. Prospective gating is mainly used in older PET systems where list mode storage is not feasible and relies on defining phases in relation to the peak of the R wave. Such phases can be defined as preceding the R wave (backward gating) or occurring after it (forward gating). In both scenarios, the annihilation events can be sorted into predefined sinogram buffers and reconstructed once the acquisition is completed.

Cardiac gating can serve 2 functions: (1) it can be used for motion compensation of the myocardium[35] and (2) it can be used for functional assessment of the myocardium. The functional assessment provides both diagnostic and prognostic value in the clinical assessment of global cardiac function (left ventricular ejection fraction, LVEF), regional wall motion abnormalities, and myocardial dyssynchrony.[36,37] The motion-compensated images are mainly used for research purposes, whereas the functional assessments are used in the clinical routine. Analyses of the functional parameters have shown that an increase in LVEF (from baseline to peak stress) is inversely related to the magnitude of ischemia and the extent of angiographic CAD.[38,39] In patients with multivessel CAD, LVEF often shows a blunted response or can even drop on stress imaging. The change in LVEF during peak stress has been shown to have value for risk prediction.[40,41] In addition, cardiac gating has been proven a strong tool as a first approach in the assessment in the coronary plaques because the coronary arteries can shift up to 26 mm during the cardiac cycle[32,42,43] (**Fig. 2**).

RESPIRATORY GATING

Respiratory gating is desired in the clinical settings to improve image quality but is not often used in many modern systems, which only allow for one form of gating during the reconstruction (ECG or respiratory gating). In systems facilitating dual-physiological trigger events (cardiorespiratory signals), the respiratory signal may be extracted using external markers such as piezo-electric respiratory belts or infrared systems.[24] Other solutions using spirometers, and measurements of the nasal temperature/humidity have also been successfully tested.[44] Respiratory gating using external

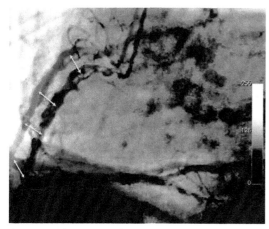

Fig. 2. Displacement of the coronary arteries during the cardiac contraction. The coronary arteries are shifting 8 to 26 mm during cardiac contraction (*arrows*).

markers has several drawbacks. These drawbacks include a time-consuming imaging setup,[45] potential malfunction during the acquisition,[46] and rather rigid monitoring of the respiratory signal, which results in less robust monitoring in patients with changes in the respiratory baseline.[47] Owing to the complex setups, the introduction of respiratory gating is still mainly a tool applied in research studies primarily in centers with technical personnel who can maintain the systems.

To overcome the drawbacks of the external markers, the tendency in recent research is to replace the external markers using data-driven methods.[34] The data-driven methods offer several benefits over the use of external markers: First, the data-driven methods do not require frequent calibrations because they extract the respiratory signal directly from the PET list files.[45] Second, they allow for ad hoc correction of all scans acquired in list mode format, whereas careful planning is needed when using external markers. A third benefit is that the data-driven methods do not require the user to buy any additional hardware, which can be costly to both acquire and install.

In addition, the data-driven methods, in general, have the potential of facilitating accurate gating in patients with changes in the respiratory baseline, a frequent problem in myocardial perfusion imaging, where stress scans are performed after administration of pharmaceutical agents. The common agents (Adenosine, Dipyridamole, and Regadenoson) all have short half-lives, which require optimized stressing protocols such that the maximum effect is obtained during the infusion of the PET tracer. Given the fast roll-off effect of the

pharmaceuticals, it is not uncommon to encounter changes in the respiratory baseline during the acquisition.[48,49] If not corrected for, the change in the respiratory baseline might introduce a degradation of the gated images in comparison to the nongated images.[50] Here, data-driven gating approaches allow for tailored gating approaches that fit the stress-imaging protocol and thus have the potential of outperforming the use of the external markers, which often are calibrated to the respiratory baseline at the beginning of the acquisition.[47,51]

Sensitivity-based Methods

The first attempts at extracting information of the respiratory motion directly from the PET-raw data (list files) were proposed by Bundschuh and colleagues[52] and He and colleagues.[53] These methods, in brief, are based on the heterogeneous sensitivity profiles that exist in all PET systems. The sensitivity profile is partly introduced by the geometry of the system and partly by the detector materials used.[54] Owing to the geometry in the PET system, the highest sensitivity is obtained in the center of the field of view. Heterogeneous objects moving in and out of the center field of view will result in changes in the obtained count rates equivalent to the motion in the scanners axial direction. For patient scans, the heterogeneous uptake rates are obtained through differences in the tracer distribution as well as differences in the linear attenuation coefficients in the lungs and diaphragm.

Center-of-Mass/Centroid-of-Mass–based Methods

The center-of-mass or centroid-of-mass (CoM)-based approaches have gained substantial interest in imaging of organs with focal uptake and high contrast to background ratio, such as myocardial scans, and in studies of non–small cell lung cancers. Several methods relying on this assessment have been proposed, using either the full field of view or through detection of localized motion vector fields.[44,55] The CoM assessment, in brief, evaluates the centroid of the counts obtained in the region of interest using single-slice rebinned sinograms (SSRB).[56] The SSRB algorithm, in short, is an algorithm that compresses the full 3D sinograms into a reduced 3D sinogram. By performing the compression, the noise is reduced and felicitates extraction of more stable respiratory signal.

Sinogram Fluctuation Model

The sinogram fluctuation model evaluates the fluctuations obtained in sinograms with short time duration (~500 ms). Following their binning, the sinograms can be evaluated for the periodicity of the signal changes in each of the short time-duration datasets, thus permitting extraction of the respiratory signal using only data with frequencies within the normal respiratory range (2- to 9-second periodicity).[57]

MR-based Approaches

The introduction of the hybrid PET/MR systems has facilitated new methods for motion detection, in which accurate estimates of the respiratory signal can be extracted directly from the diaphragm in the PET images.[58–61] The respiratory signal can be obtained either from dedicated MR sequences that target the golden angle[58] or through tracking of the heart/diaphragm in standard MR sequences.[60] The resulting data can be used either for respiratory gating or for motion compensation during the image reconstruction.[29,58] Despite the accurate tracking of both respiratory and cardiac motion through dedicated MR sequences, the MR-based approaches have some drawbacks. They can only be used in integrated PET/MR systems and often require specific MR sequences for motion detection, which can limit the time left for the acquisition of clinically important data.[58]

Respiratory gating: phase versus amplitude

Once acquired, the respiratory signal can be used for gating in multiple ways, where phase-based/time-based (similar to the ECG-based gating approaches) and amplitude-based gating are the two most common approaches (**Fig. 3**).[51]

Time-based/phase-based gating The phase-based method is the most simplistic method of the two, where each respiratory phase is divided into a user-defined number of phases, each with equal time duration.[51] The equal duration of the gates ensures homogeneous noise levels for all gates, which is beneficial in the subsequent analyses. Unfortunately, this method does not allow for differentiating between normal tidal breathing and sudden excessive in/expiratory breath-holds or changes in the respiratory baseline.

Amplitude-based gating The amplitude-based gating offers more accurate gating than the time-based/phase-based gating approach. Despite the superiority in providing high-spatial differentiation of data from different respiratory amplitudes, this technique also has its limitations. The highly dynamic range of respiratory signals often hampers its functionality and thus most often requires truncation or discarding of data outside the normal range to ensure enough counts to provide images with diagnostic quality. In addition, the asynchronous respiratory cycle will often introduce inhomogeneities in the noise characteristics in the resulting gated images with the best quality often obtained in the end-expiratory phase. Because of this, it has been proposed to use the optimal respiratory gate, which only uses data from the end-expiratory phase, known as the optimal respiratory phase, which typically can contain up to 35% of all image counts.[62]

DUAL GATING

The single gating techniques have been proven suboptimal for many PET scans because the remaining motion pattern is still embedded in the resulting images. Dual-gating approaches, which

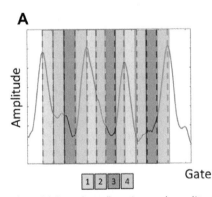
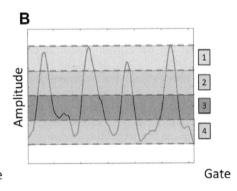

Fig. 3. Time-based (phase-based) gating and amplitude-based gating techniques, here exemplified using 4 respiratory gates. (*A*) Time-based method divides the data into equally time-divided bins that will have the same noise properties (equal time duration). (*B*) Amplitude-based gating divides the data into bins with the same respiratory amplitude and thereby poses the risk of having different count rates in gates, as can be observed for the third respiratory cycle, which does not reach the same amplitude as the preceding cycles.

combine the cardiorespiratory motion, have been proposed.[26,63–65] The combination of the two gating techniques ensures virtually motion-free images, with only little intragate motion present (**Fig. 4**). Unfortunately, this requires sufficient image quality (count rates per single gate) in the subsequent reconstructions, as often up to 16 to 64 gates are being used. The exact number depends on how many respiratory and cardiac gates are used ($N_{Respiratory}$ gates $\times$ $N_{cardiac}$ gates),[66,67] with N being the number of the respective gates.

PET ATTENUATION CORRECTION ISSUES RESULTING FROM MOTION

Attenuation correction (AC) is an important prerequisite for absolute quantification in PET imaging. Several AC techniques have been proposed, depending on the modality (PET only, PET/CT, or PET/MR).[68–70] Several drawbacks and limitations have been described for the AC techniques. The drawbacks include both physiologic and technical aspects, such as beam-hardening, misalignment, truncation as well as nonphysiological artifacts. In the context of gating, especially the misalignment artifacts are particularly relevant. The remaining artifacts have a more general character and have been discussed thoroughly elsewhere.[71,72]

Misalignment of the PET emission data and the AC images can be classified as either repositioning events where the patient moves between the acquisition of the AC maps and the PET-emission data, differences between the respiratory-gated PET-images and the corresponding AC maps, or as breathing during the AC acquisition (**Fig. 5**).[73–75]

Respiratory motion during the PET images translates the heart by up to a few centimeters (see section Respiratory gating). Because of the fast acquisition times of the AC images (a few seconds in CT, 30 seconds in PET/MR systems), respiratory motion during the acquisition is often not a problem regardless of whether a free-breathing or end-expiratory breath-hold acquisition protocol is used.[76] Several optimizations of AC acquisitions have been proposed for both the PET/MR and the PET/CT systems. Using cine CT for PET/CT has been suggested.[77] From the cine CT, it is possible to reconstruct a respiratory-averaged AC map with the same displacements as obtained during the cine CT acquisition. In PET/MR systems, it has been proposed to acquire several AC maps in different respiratory positions because

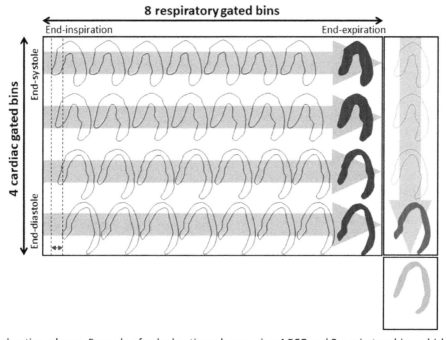

Fig. 4. Dual-gating scheme. Example of a dual gating scheme using 4 ECG and 8 respiratory bins, which creates a total of 32 virtually motion-free images. Each of the gated images can be coregistered to obtain images with reduced noise properties when compared with the noise in each individual gate. This research was originally published in *Journal of Nuclear Medicine*. (*Data from* Slomka PJ, Rubeaux M, Le Meunier L, et al. Dual-gated motion-frozen cardiac PET with flurpiridaz F 18. J Nucl Med 2015;56(12):1876–81. © SNMMI.)

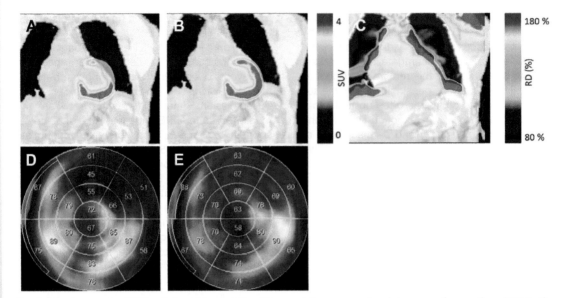

Fig. 5. Displacement of PET emission data and the AC maps (*A*) can cause local changes of more than 80% in the quantitative assessment (*B, C*). Correction for the misalignment of the AC maps and PET data reduced the extent and severity of the hypometabolic region (*D, E*). The displacements can be introduced through respiratory motion during the PET acquisition or by patient repositioning between the acquisition of the AC map and the PET data. This figure was originally published in *Journal of Nuclear Cardiology* under the Creative Commons Attribution 4.0 International License (http://creativecommons.org/licenses/by/4.0/). (*Data from* Lassen ML, Rasul S, Beitzke D, et al. Assessment of attenuation correction for myocardial PET imaging using combined PET/MRI. J Nucl Cardiol 2017:1–12 © The Author(s) 2017.)

the AC images are acquired without the use of ionizing radiation.

NEW GATING TECHNIQUES AND CHALLENGES AHEAD

Cardiorespiratory motion has been investigated by many researchers, and several gating approaches have been proposed. The use of external markers has been used in the conventional assessment of the displacement during the acquisition. However, recent trends indicate that data-driven gating techniques are an emerging technology that will permit markerless motion detection in clinical routine. These gating techniques mainly focus on respiratory motion detection, although cardiac gating might also be possible as demonstrated for the first time in 2009.[34,44] Although these established techniques might replace conventional external marker methods, the potential of data-driven detection of patient repositioning events is another interesting field of research. A recent pilot study has shown that such techniques are feasible in coronary plaque studies, in which gross patient motion has a detrimental effect on the quantitative accuracy.[78] Furthermore, it is thought that tracer-kinetic studies for novel PET tracers, where scanning protocols can last up to 1 hour or more, will benefit from patient repositioning detection,

ultimately enabling triple-gating or application of sophisticated combinations of various gating techniques.[79]

Moreover, the use of gated images is expected to be implemented in motion compensation techniques, either during or before image reconstruction. Utilizing non-image based motion compensation will improve the image quality of the static images, where accurate definition of pathophysiologic changes can be difficult in the gated images due to the increased noise levels. By correcting for the motion during image reconstruction, it is possible to obtain a fully motion-compensated image with the spatial resolution similar to gated images, with the noise characteristics of the static image acquisitions. In addition, the motion-compensated images can also reduce the respiratory blur in the ECG-gated reconstructions and thus lead to improved quantification of left ventricular volumes for function assessments. Therefore, gating will become increasingly important in the future not only for the detection of motion but also in the pursuit of accurate assessment of physiologic parameters.

SUMMARY

In this article, gating approaches for both cardiac and respiratory motion have been reviewed.

Cardiac gating has enabled accurate heart and coronary imaging whereas respiratory gating has become an important frontier in PET imaging. With multiple limitations of currently used external marker methods and the increasing availability of list mode PET data, the field is now moving toward data-driven techniques, as a promising alternative. Ultimately, dual gating encompassing both cardiac and respiratory motion or even triple gating, which also takes into account gross patient motion effects, shall lead to further improvements in image quality.

REFERENCES

1. Bengel FM, Higuchi T, Javadi MS, et al. Cardiac positron emission tomography. J Am Coll Cardiol 2009;54(1):1–15.

2. Di Carli MF, Dorbala S, Meserve J, et al. Clinical myocardial perfusion PET/CT. J Nucl Med 2007; 48(5):783–93.

3. Bateman TM, Dilsizian V, Beanlands RS, et al. American Society of Nuclear Cardiology and Society of Nuclear Medicine and Molecular Imaging Joint Position Statement on the clinical indications for myocardial perfusion PET. J Nucl Med 2016;57(10):1654–6.

4. Kong EJ, Lee SH, Cho IH. Myocardial fibrosis in hypertrophic cardiomyopathy demonstrated by integrated cardiac F-18 FDG PET/MR. Nucl Med Mol Imaging 2013;47(3):196–200.

5. Bravo PE, Di Carli MF, Dorbala S. Role of PET to evaluate coronary microvascular dysfunction in non-ischemic cardiomyopathies. Heart Fail Rev 2017;22(4):455–64.

6. Skali H, Schulman AR, Dorbala S. 18F-FDG PET/CT for the assessment of myocardial sarcoidosis. Curr Cardiol Rep 2013;15(4):352.

7. Hulten E, Aslam S, Osborne M, et al. Cardiac sarcoidosis-state of the art review. Cardiovasc Diagn Ther 2016;6(1):50–63.

8. Dorbala S, Vangala D, Semer J, et al. Imaging cardiac amyloidosis: a pilot study using 18F-florbetapir positron emission tomography. Eur J Nucl Med Mol Imaging 2014;41(9):1652–62.

9. Sarrazin JF, Philippon F, Tessier M, et al. Usefulness of fluorine-18 positron emission tomography/computed tomography for identification of cardiovascular implantable electronic device infections. J Am Coll Cardiol 2012;59(18):1616–25.

10. Kim J, Feller ED, Chen W, et al. FDG PET/CT for early detection and localization of left ventricular assist device infection. impact on patient management and outcome. JACC Cardiovasc Imaging 2018; 1–8. https://doi.org/10.1016/j.jcmg.2018.01.024.

11. Dweck MR, Chow MWL, Joshi NV, et al. Coronary arterial 18F-sodium fluoride uptake: a novel marker of plaque biology. J Am Coll Cardiol 2012;59(17): 1539–48.

12. Joshi NV, Vesey AT, Williams MC, et al. 18F-fluoride positron emission tomography for identification of ruptured and high-risk coronary atherosclerotic plaques: a prospective clinical trial. Lancet 2014; 383(9918):705–13.

13. Kwiecinski J, Adamson PD, Lassen ML, et al. Feasibility of Coronary 18F-Sodium Fluoride Positron-Emission Tomography Assessment With the Utilization of Previously Acquired Computed Tomography Angiography. Circ Cardiovasc Imaging 2018; 11(12):e008325.

14. Hacker M. Monitoring anti-inflammatory therapies in patients with atherosclerosis: FDG PET emerges as the method of choice. Eur J Nucl Med Mol Imaging 2012;39(3):396–8.

15. Rahmim A, Rousset O, Zaidi H. Strategies for motion tracking and correction in PET. PET Clin 2007;2(2): 251–66.

16. Cal-Gonzalez J, Rausch I, Sundar LKS, et al. Hybrid imaging: instrumentation and data processing. Front Phys 2018;6. https://doi.org/10.3389/fphy.2018. 00047.

17. Conti M. Focus on time-of-flight PET: the benefits of improved time resolution. Eur J Nucl Med Mol Imaging 2011;38(6):1147–57.

18. Dasari PKR, Jones JP, Casey ME, et al. The effect of time-of-flight and point spread function modeling on 82Rb myocardial perfusion imaging of obese patients. J Nucl Cardiol 2018. https://doi.org/10.1007/ s12350-018-1311-y.

19. Slomka PJ, Pan T, Berman DS, et al. Advances in SPECT and PET hardware. Prog Cardiovasc Dis 2015;57(6):566–78.

20. Armstrong IS, Tonge CM, Arumugam P. Impact of point spread function modeling and time-of-flight on myocardial blood flow and myocardial flow reserve measurements for rubidium-82 cardiac PET. J Nucl Cardiol 2014;21(3):467–74.

21. Rubeaux M, Doris MK, Alessio A, et al. Enhancing cardiac PET by motion correction techniques. Curr Cardiol Rep 2017;19(2). https://doi.org/10.1007/ s11886-017-0825-2.

22. Blankstein R, Osborne M, Naya M, et al. Cardiac positron emission tomography enhances prognostic assessments of patients with suspected cardiac sarcoidosis. J Am Coll Cardiol 2014;63(4):329–36.

23. Nensa F, Bamberg F, Rischpler C, et al. Hybrid cardiac imaging using PET/MRI: a joint position statement by the European Society of Cardiovascular Radiology (ESCR) and the European Association of Nuclear Medicine (EANM). Eur Radiol 2018;1–16. https://doi.org/10.1007/s00330-017-5008-4.

24. Nehmeh SA, Erdi YE. Respiratory motion in positron emission tomography/computed tomography: a review. Semin Nucl Med 2008;38(3):167–76.

25. Ter-Pogossian MM, Bergmann SR, Sobel BE. Influence of cardiac and respiratory motion on tomographic reconstructions of the heart: implications for quantitative nuclear cardiology. J Comput Assist Tomogr 1982;6(6):1148–55. Available at: http://www.ncbi.nlm.nih.gov/pubmed/6983534.

26. Teras M, Kokki T, Durand-Schaefer N, et al. Dual-gated cardiac PET-Clinical feasibility study. Eur J Nucl Med Mol Imaging 2010;37(3):505–16.

27. Rubeaux M, Joshi NV, Dweck MR, et al. Motion correction of 18F-NaF PET for imaging coronary atherosclerotic plaques. J Nucl Med 2016;57(1):54–9.

28. Chander A, Brenner M, Lautamäki R, et al. Comparison of measures of left ventricular function from electrocardiographically gated 82 Rb PET with contrast-enhanced CT ventriculography: a hybrid PET/CT analysis. J Nucl Med 2008;49:1643–50.

29. Manber R, Thielemans K, Hutton BF, et al. Joint PET-MR respiratory motion models for clinical PET motion correction. Phys Med Biol 2016;61(17):6515.

30. Thielemans K, Schleyer P, Marsden PK, et al. Data-driven dual-gating for cardiac PET. In: 2014 IEEE Nuclear Science Symposium and Medical Imaging Conference (NSS/MIC). Seattle (WA), November 8-15, 2014.

31. Dawood M, Büther F, Stegger L, et al. Optimal number of respiratory gates in positron emission tomography: a cardiac patient study. Med Phys 2009;36(5):1775–84.

32. Shechter G, Resar JR, McVeigh ER. Displacement and velocity of the coronary arteries: cardiac and respiratory motion. IEEE Trans Med Imaging 2006;25(3):369–75. Available at: http://www.ncbi.nlm.nih.gov/pmc/articles/PMC2396264/.

33. Nekolla SG, Dinges J, Rischpler C. Clinical impact of cardiac-gated PET imaging. PET Clin 2013;8(1):69–79.

34. Kesner AL, Schleyer PJ, Büther F, et al. On transcending the impasse of respiratory motion correction applications in routine clinical imaging – a consideration of a fully automated data driven motion control framework. EJNMMI Phys 2014;1(1):8.

35. Le Meunier L, Slomka PJ, Dey D, et al. Motion frozen 18F-FDG cardiac PET. J Nucl Cardiol 2011;18(2):259–66.

36. Pazhenkottil AP, Buechel RR, Nkoulou R, et al. Left ventricular dyssynchrony assessment by phase analysis from gated PET-FDG scans. J Nucl Cardiol 2011;18(5):920–5.

37. AlJaroudi W, Alraies MC, Hachamovitch R, et al. Association of left ventricular mechanical dyssynchrony with survival benefit from revascularization: a study of gated positron emission tomography in patients with ischemic LV dysfunction and narrow QRS. Eur J Nucl Med Mol Imaging 2012;39(10):1581–91.

38. Dorbala S, Vangala D, Sampson U, et al. Value of vasodilator left ventricular ejection fraction reserve in evaluating the magnitude of myocardium at risk and the extent of angiographic coronary artery disease: a 82Rb PET/CT study. J Nucl Med 2007;48(3):349–58.

39. Brown TLY, Merrill J, Volokh L, et al. Determinants of the response of left ventricular ejection fraction to vasodilator stress in electrocardiographically gated 82rubidium myocardial perfusion PET. Eur J Nucl Med Mol Imaging 2008;35(2):336–42.

40. Lertsburapa K, Ahlberg A, Bateman T, et al. Independent and incremental prognostic value of left ventricular ejection fraction determined by stress gated rubidium 82 PET imaging in patients with known or suspected coronary artery disease. J Nucl Cardiol 2008;15(6):745–53.

41. Dorbala S, Hachamovitch R, Curillova Z, et al. Incremental prognostic value of gated Rb-82 positron emission tomography myocardial perfusion imaging over clinical variables and rest LVEF. JACC Cardiovasc Imaging 2009;2(7):846–54.

42. Dilsizian V, Bacharach SL, Beanlands RS, et al. ASNC imaging guidelines/SNMMI procedure standard for positron emission tomography (PET) nuclear cardiology procedures. J Nucl Cardiol 2016;23. https://doi.org/10.1007/s12350-016-0522-3.

43. Rubeaux M, Joshi N, Dweck MR, et al. Demons versus level-set motion registration for coronary 18 F-sodium fluoride PET. Proc SPIE Int Soc Opt Eng 2016. https://doi.org/10.1117/12.2217179.

44. Büther F, Dawood M, Stegger L, et al. List mode-driven cardiac and respiratory gating in PET. J Nucl Med 2009;50(5):674–81.

45. Giraud P, Houle A. Respiratory gating for radiotherapy: main technical aspects and clinical benefits. Bull Cancer 2010;97(7):847–56 [in French].

46. Liu C, Pierce LA II, Alessio AM, et al. The impact of respiratory motion on tumor quantification and delineation in static PET/CT imaging. Phys Med Biol 2009;54(24):7345.

47. Lassen ML, Rasmussen T, Christensen TE, et al. Respiratory gating in cardiac PET: effects of adenosine and dipyridamole. J Nucl Cardiol 2016. https://doi.org/10.1007/s12350-016-0631-z.

48. Memmott MJ, Tonge CM, Saint KJ, et al. Impact of pharmacological stress agent on patient motion during rubidium-82 myocardial perfusion PET/CT. J Nucl Cardiol 2017;1–10. https://doi.org/10.1007/s12350-016-0767-x.

49. Watt A, Routledge P. Adenosine stimulates respiration in man. Br J Clin Pharmacol 1985;20(5):503–6.

50. Gould KL. Optimizing quantitative myocardial perfusion by positron emission tomography for guiding CAD management. J Nucl Cardiol 2016. https://doi.org/10.1007/s12350-016-0666-1.

51. Dawood M, Buther F, Lang N, et al. Respiratory gating in positron emission tomography: a quantitative comparison of different gating schemes. Med Phys 2007;34(7):3067–76.

52. Bundschuh RA, Martínez-Moeller A, Essler M, et al. Postacquisition detection of tumor motion in the lung and upper abdomen using list-mode PET data: a feasibility study. J Nucl Med 2007;48(5):758–63.

53. He J, O'Keefe GJ, Gong SJ, et al. A novel method for respiratory motion gated with geometric sensitivity of the scanner in 3D PET. IEEE Trans Nucl Sci 2008;55(5):2557–65.

54. Eriksson L, Townsend D, Conti M, et al. An investigation of sensitivity limits in PET scanners. Nucl Instrum Methods Phys Res A 2007;580(2):836–42.

55. Büther F, Ernst I, Dawood M, et al. Detection of respiratory tumour motion using intrinsic list mode-driven gating in positron emission tomography. Eur J Nucl Med Mol Imaging 2010;37(12):2315–27.

56. Daube-Witherspoon ME, Muehllehner G. Treatment of axial data in three-dimensional PET. J Nucl Med 1987;28(11):1717–24. Available at: http://www.ncbi.nlm.nih.gov/pubmed/3499493.

57. Kesner AL, Kuntner C. A new fast and fully automated software based algorithm for extracting respiratory signal from raw PET data and its comparison to other methods. Med Phys 2010;37(10):5550–9.

58. Grimm R, Fürst S, Souvatzoglou M, et al. Self-gated MRI motion modeling for respiratory motion compensation in integrated PET/MRI. Med Image Anal 2014;19(1):110–20.

59. Munoz C, Kolbitsch C, Reader AJ, et al. MR-based cardiac and respiratory motion-compensation techniques for PET-MR imaging. PET Clin 2016;11(2):179–91.

60. Munoz C, Neji R, Cruz G, et al. Motion-corrected simultaneous cardiac positron emission tomography and coronary MR angiography with high acquisition efficiency. Magn Reson Med 2018;79(1):339–50.

61. Munoz C, Kunze KP, Neji R, et al. Motion-corrected whole-heart PET-MR for the simultaneous visualisation of coronary artery integrity and myocardial viability: an initial clinical validation. Eur J Nucl Med Mol Imaging 2018. https://doi.org/10.1007/s00259-018-4047-7.

62. Liu C, Alessio A, Pierce L, et al. Quiescent period respiratory gating for PET/CT. Med Phys 2010;37(9):5037–43.

63. Gigengack F, Ruthotto L, Burger M, et al. Motion correction in dual gated cardiac PET using mass-preserving image registration. IEEE Trans Med Imaging 2012;31(3):698–712.

64. Lamare F, Le Maitre A, Dawood M, et al. Evaluation of respiratory and cardiac motion correction schemes in dual gated PET/CT cardiac imaging. Med Phys 2014;41(7):072504.

65. Hyun MC, Gerlach J, Rubeaux M, et al. Technical consideration for dual ECG/respiratory-gated cardiac PET imaging. J Nucl Cardiol 2017;24(4):1246–52.

66. Slomka PJ, Rubeaux M, Le Meunier L, et al. Dual-gated motion-frozen cardiac PET with flurpiridaz F18. J Nucl Med 2015;56(12):1876–81.

67. Martinez-Möller A, Zikic D, Botnar RM, et al. Dual cardiac-respiratory gated PET: implementation and results from a feasibility study. Eur J Nucl Med Mol Imaging 2007;34(9):1447–54.

68. Chesler DA. 3-Dimensional activity distribution from multiple positron scintigraphs. J Nucl Med 1971;12:347.

69. Kinahan PE, Hasegawa BH, Beyer T. X-ray-based attenuation correction for positron emission tomography/computed tomography scanners. Semin Nucl Med 2003;33(3):166–79.

70. Martinez-Möller A, Souvatzoglou M, Delso G, et al. Tissue classification as a potential approach for attenuation correction in whole-body PET/MRI: evaluation with PET/CT data. J Nucl Med 2009;50(4):520–6.

71. Sureshbabu W, Mawlawi O. PET/CT imaging artifacts. J Nucl Med Technol 2005;33(200218):156–61. Available at: http://interactive.snm.org/docs/JNMT_Exam_PETCT_Imaging_Artifacts.pdf.

72. Keller SH, Holm S, Hansen AE, et al. Image artifacts from MR-based attenuation correction in clinical, whole-body PET/MRI. MAGMA 2013;26(1):173–81.

73. Martinez-Möller A, Souvatzoglou M, Navab N, et al. Artifacts from misaligned CT in cardiac perfusion solutions. J Nucl Med 2007;48(2):188–94.

74. Gould KL, Pan T, Loghin C, et al. Frequent diagnostic errors in cardiac PET/CT due to misregistration of CT attenuation and emission PET images: a definitive analysis of causes, consequences, and corrections. J Nucl Med 2007;48(7):1112–21.

75. Lassen ML, Rasul S, Beitzke D, et al. Assessment of attenuation correction for myocardial PET imaging using combined PET/MRI. J Nucl Cardiol 2017;1–12. https://doi.org/10.1007/s12350-017-1118-2.

76. Beyer T, Lassen ML, Boellaard R, et al. Investigating the state-of-the-art in whole-body MR-based attenuation correction: an intra-individual, inter-system, inventory study on three clinical PET/MR systems. MAGMA 2016;29(1):75–87.

77. Pan T, Mawlawi O, Luo D, et al. Attenuation correction of PET cardiac data with low-dose average CT in PET/CT. Med Phys 2006;33(10):3931–8.

78. Lassen ML, Kwiecinski J, Cadet S, et al. Data-driven gross patient motion detection and compensation: Implications for coronary ^{18}F-NaF PET imaging. J Nucl Med 2018. [Epub ahead of print].

79. Piccinelli M, Votaw JR, Garcia EV. Motion correction and its impact on absolute myocardial blood flow measures with PET. Curr Cardiol Rep 2018;20(5). https://doi.org/10.1007/s11886-018-0977-8.

Potential Role of PET in Assessing Ventricular Arrhythmias

Daniele Muser, MD[a], Simon A. Castro, MD[a],
Abass Alavi, MD, MD (Hon), PhD (Hon), DSc (Hon)[b],
Pasquale Santangeli, MD, PhD[a],*

KEYWORDS

• Ventricular arrhythmias • Positron emission tomography • Cardiomyopathy • Inflammation

KEY POINTS

• Ventricular arrhythmias (VAs) are a major cause of morbidity and mortality, especially in patients with structural heart disease, and the detailed characterization of the underlying substrate is pivotal in terms of risk stratification and management.
• PET imaging offers a valuable tool to characterize different aspects of the arrhythmogenic substrate by evaluating myocardial perfusion, presence of inflammation, viability, and sympathetic innervation with different radiotracers.
• Myocardial inflammation plays a central role in the genesis and maintenance of VAs determining irreversible cell damage with scar formation, constituting the substrate for reentrant arrhythmias, but also with functional mechanisms like triggered activity and exacerbated automaticity within inflamed areas.
• ^{18}F-fluorodeoxyglucose-PET allows detection of both active inflammation and scar, which has demonstrated to be of great diagnostic, prognostic, and therapeutic value in patients with VAs.
• Ongoing areas of research include the use of PET to identify sites of abnormal myocardial sympathetic innervation as a source of VAs and potential target of interventional procedures.

INTRODUCTION

Ventricular arrhythmias (VAs) have a wide range of clinical manifestations, ranging from mildly symptomatic frequent premature ventricular contractions (PVCs) to life-threatening events, such as sustained ventricular tachycardia (VT) or ventricular fibrillation (VF). Myocardial scar plays a central role in the genesis and maintenance of reentrant arrhythmias, which are commonly associated with structural heart disease, such as ischemic heart disease, healed myocarditis, and nonischemic cardiomyopathies. However, the arrhythmogenic substrate may remain unclear in up to 50% of the cases after routine diagnostic workup.[1,2] In this setting, there is growing evidence that clinically unrecognized myocardial inflammation may play a role in patients presenting with arrhythmias of unexplained origin.[1] Not only active myocardial inflammation may lead to myocyte loss and reparative fibrosis representing the ideal milieu of reentrant arrhythmias but also inflammation may alter the electrophysiological properties of myocardial cells, leading to various forms of arrhythmias.[3] In the last decade, cardiac PET/computed tomography (CT) imaging has acquired a growing role in the identification and characterization of myocardial arrhythmogenic substrate, providing information

Conflict of Interest: The authors have no disclosures.
[a] Cardiac Electrophysiology, Cardiovascular Medicine Division, Hospital of the University of Pennsylvania, 3400 Spruce Street, Philadelphia, PA 19104, USA; [b] Nuclear Medicine Division, Radiology Department, Hospital of the University of Pennsylvania, 3400 Spruce Street, Philadelphia, PA 19104, USA
* Corresponding author.
E-mail address: pasquale.santangeli@uphs.upenn.edu

pet.theclinics.com

about the presence of myocardial inflammation, which may otherwise remain unrecognized.[4,5] Moreover, PET/CT has recently demonstrated to be of great value in evaluating treatment response in order to improve long-term outcomes.[6,7] Other applications of PET imaging include identification of areas of abnormal myocardial perfusion, metabolism, and innervation, which all may be involved in the genesis and maintenance of VAs and represent potential targets for catheter ablation (CA). In the present article, the authors review the available data regarding the utility of PET/CT in the workup of VAs with a special focus on its prognostic relevance and its application in planning and guiding interventional treatments.

PATHOPHYSIOLOGY

Inflammation contributes to the development of VAs in both a direct and an indirect way.[3] Active inflammation inevitably determines myocardial structural changes related to direct cell injury and replacement fibrosis. The coexistence of surviving myocardial fibers within scarred tissue leads to the formation of slow conduction pathways as well as to a dispersion of activation and refractoriness able to sustain reentrant circuits.[8] On the counterpart, systemic release of inflammatory cytokines, such as tumor necrosis factor alpha, interleukin-1, and interleukin-6, is involved in electrical remodeling of myocardial cells by changing the expression and function of potassium and calcium channels as well as determining a sympathetic activation of the central nervous system, which all together promote myocardial electrical instability and contribute to generate VAs.[9] Moreover, myocardial ischemia resulting from microvascular and macrovascular dysfunction within the inflamed myocardium can further increase its arrhythmogenicity.[10] Various PET/CT scan modalities, using different radiolabel tracers conjugated with metabolically active molecules, are able to target the different pathophysiologic aspects of arrhythmogenicity, such as identification of areas of inducible ischemia with ^{11}C-acetate, ^{13}N-ammonia, ^{15}O-water, and [82]Rb, detection of active inflammation and distinction between scar and viable tissue with ^{18}F-fluorodeoxyglucose (^{18}F-FDG), and evaluation of sympathetic innervation with ^{11}C-hydroxyephedrine (^{11}C-HED).

PREVALENCE AND CHARACTERIZATION OF MYOCARDIAL INFLAMMATION IN PATIENTS WITH VENTRICULAR ARRHYTHMIAS OF UNKNOWN CAUSE

Few studies have investigated the potential role of subclinical myocardial inflammation in determining

VAs. Tung and colleagues[1] have evaluated the prevalence of abnormal ^{18}F-FDG uptake in a series of 103 patients presenting with VAs (14% with frequent PVCs, 81% with sustained VT, and 5% with resuscitated VF) in the setting of nonischemic cardiomyopathy of unknown cause. They applied a rigorous ^{18}F-FDG-PET/CT acquisition protocol with at least 16 hours of fasting before full body and dedicated myocardial ^{18}F-FDG uptake images acquisition in order to suppress physiologic ^{18}F-FDG uptake by myocardial cells and enhance abnormal ^{18}F-FDG uptake by activated macrophages. In order to identify perfusion abnormalities, myocardial perfusion at rest was also assessed with intravenous ^{13}N-ammonia 1 hour before intravenous administration of ^{18}F-FDG. To increase the specificity of PET results, only patients presenting focal or focal on diffuse patterns of myocardial ^{18}F-FDG uptake were considered PET positive and classified into 4 groups based on evidence of extracardiac abnormal ^{18}F-FDG uptake and perfusion abnormalities (early stage in the absence of perfusion abnormalities vs late stage if focal perfusion defects were present). Almost 50% of the patients (50 out of 103) had evidence of abnormal myocardial ^{18}F-FDG uptake with signs of extracardiac involvement in 34% of them. In the subgroup of patients in whom an endomyocardial biopsy (EMB) was performed, nongranulomatous inflammation was found in 30% of the cases, whereas cardiac sarcoidosis (CS) was found in 60% and absence of inflammatory infiltrates was found in the remaining 10% of them. Of note, one patient underwent cardiac transplantation, and pathologic examination of the explanted heart revealed focal nonnecrotizing granulomas; this patient had positive ^{18}F-FDG-PET, but 2 negative EMBs. Among patients treated with CA, a correlation between ^{18}F-FDG-PET findings and voltage abnormalities was reported in 79% of the cases. Immunosuppressive treatment was started in 90% of patients with positive ^{18}F-FDG-PET/CT. Patients with early-stage disease had a trend toward better clinical outcomes compared with those with late-stage disease (VT-free survival 72% vs 56%, respectively). Based on the above results, the investigators hypothesized that concealed myocardial inflammation may play a role in the genesis of VAs in a nonnegligible proportion of patients otherwise considered "idiopathic." These patients may benefit from early detection of the underlying disease (before irreversible myocardial scarring occurs) and from immunosuppressive medical therapy.[1] Those findings have recently been confirmed and expanded by a single-center prospective study (MAVERIC, Myocarditis And

Ventricular Arrhythmia registry) in which ^{18}F-FDG-PET was performed in a series of 107 patients with frequent (≥5000/24 h) PVCs of unexplained cause following at least 18 hours of fasting preceded by 24 hours of high-fat-content diet.[11] As previously reported, only focal or focal on diffuse myocardial ^{18}F-FDG uptake patterns were considered significant. Patients with positive ^{18}F-FDG-PET were treated with immunosuppressive therapy (oral prednisone 40 mg daily tapered 10 mg every 3 weeks for a total of 3 months). In patients who had either a suboptimal or no response at 3 months, a second-line immunosuppressive treatment with azathioprine, cyclosporine, mycophenolate, methotrexate, or monoclonal antibodies was considered. ^{18}F-FDG-PET scans were repeated every 3 months in order to monitor treatment response and modify therapy. At baseline, 51% of the patients had evidence of abnormal myocardial ^{18}F-FDG uptake, and EMB was performed in half of them, demonstrating lymphocytic infiltrate in 46% of the cases, CS in 7%, only mild to moderate interstitial fibrosis in 25%, and no pathologic findings at all in the remaining 25% of them. Even if EMB did not show the presence of noncaseating granulomas, diagnosis of CS was made in 24% of the ^{18}F-FDG-PET–positive patients based on extracardiac findings, whereas the remaining 74% of such cases were labeled as idiopathic myocardial inflammation. A total of 46 patients received immunosuppressive treatment with optimal response (≥80% decrease in PVC burden with complete resolution of ^{18}F-FDG uptake on serial PET scans) in 67% of them, suboptimal (<80% decrease in PVC burden with only partial decrease of ^{18}F-FDG uptake) in 15%, and no response in the remaining 13% after a mean follow-up of 6 months. On the basis of these results, the investigators concluded that focal myocardial inflammation may be the cause of frequent PVCs in about half of the cases without clear cause and that ^{18}F-FDG-PET–guided immunosuppressive treatment may lead to a significant decrease of the PVC burden in most of these cases. Of note, 54% of the patients did not respond to immunosuppressive treatment, with steroids alone needing a second-line treatment.[11] The above data come from relatively small single-center experiences, are burdened by a substantial heterogeneity in treatment strategies, including CA, antiarrhythmic drugs, and type; dose and duration of immunosuppressive therapy therefore should be considered with caution: the routine application of ^{18}F-FDG-PET in patients with frequent PVCs or unexplained cardiomyopathy as well as decision to treat patients with potentially harmful immunosuppressive treatments in the absence of a specific diagnosis needs to be validated by large-scale randomized controlled studies.

ROLE OF INFLAMMATION IN PATIENTS WITH RECURRENT VENTRICULAR ARRHYTHMIAS IN THE SETTING OF CARDIAC SARCOIDOSIS AND CHAGAS DISEASE

Sarcoidosis is a systemic inflammatory disease of unknown cause characterized by lymphocyte CD4[+]-mediated formation of nonnecrotizing granulomas. Clinically overt cardiac involvement is relatively rare, being found in about 5% of the patients who may present mild clinical manifestations, such as potentially reversible AV conduction disturbances and supraventricular arrhythmias, or more severe forms characterized by recurrent VT and heart failure with progressive biventricular dysfunction.[12] Myocardial inflammation plays a central role in the genesis of VAs in CS patients by determining myocardial damage, reparative fibrosis, and scar-related reentrant arrhythmias as well as by triggered activity/exacerbated automaticity due to inflammation per se.[13,14] In this regard, a large overlap between inflammation and scar has been reported.[15,16] In candidates to VT CA, preprocedural characterization of the arrhythmogenic substrate can be useful not only for detecting potential targets for substrate-based ablation approaches but also to identify patients at high risk of recurrence that may benefit from more aggressive medical therapy with immunosuppressive drugs (Fig. 1).[7] In a series of 42 consecutive patients with CS and refractory VT referred for CA who underwent preprocedural ^{18}F-FDG-PET/CT and cardiac magnetic resonance (CMR), the authors found evidence of abnormal ^{18}F-FDG uptake in almost half (48%) of the cases, whereas areas of late gadolinium enhancement (LGE) were found in almost all (90%) the patients.[4] Interestingly, after quantification of myocardial inflammatory activity in terms of metabolic volume (MV; volume of the ^{18}F-FDG-avid myocardium) and metabolic activity (MA; product between standardized uptake value and MV), myocardial areas showing the presence of abnormal electrograms (representing potential targets for substrate-based CA) had a higher degree of scar transmurality on CMR and a lower MV and MA compared with those without evidence of abnormal electrograms (Fig. 2). Critical sites for VAs appeared more strongly associated with LGE on CMR than with increased ^{18}F-FDG uptake on PET/CT (abnormal electrograms present in 70% of LGE-positive/PET-negative myocardial segments vs 27% of LGE-negative/PET-positive

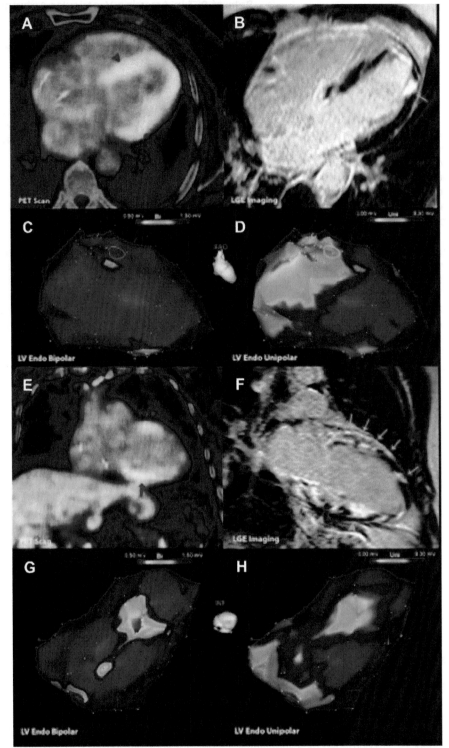

Fig. 1. Imaging and electroanatomic findings of a patient with CS and recurrent VT. PET scan (*A–E*) shows active inflammation of the midbasal inferoseptum (*A, red arrowhead*), basal (*A, asterisks*), and apical (*A, red arrow*) anterolateral wall, basal inferior (*E, red arrow*), and anterior (*E, red arrowhead*) walls. Contrast-enhanced MR imaging (*B–F*) of the same patient shows diffuse myocardial scar involving the distal anterolateral wall (*B, green arrow*), the anterior wall (*F, green arrows*), and the inferior wall (*F, green arrowheads*). The septum and the basal anterolateral wall do not show scar, although they are involved by active inflammation. Left ventricular (LV) endocardial electroanatomic map (EAM; *C, D, G,* and *H*) shows a small area of low bipolar voltage (≤1.5 mV) on the midapical inferior wall (*G, inferior view*) and a more diffuse area of low unipolar voltage (≤8.3) on the basal septum (*D, right anterior oblique [RAO] view*) and inferior wall (*H, inferior view*); unipolar EAM showed areas of abnormal voltage consistent with both scar and inflammation. (*From* Muser D, Santangeli P, Pathak RK, et al. Long-term outcomes of catheter ablation of ventricular tachycardia in patients with cardiac sarcoidosis. Circ Arrhythm Electrophysiol 2016;9:e004333; with permission.)

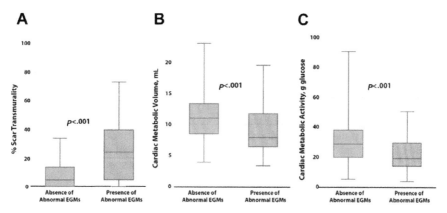

Fig. 2. MR imaging and ^{18}F-FDG-PET/CT findings according to the presence of abnormal electrograms in patients with CS and recurrent VT. Box-plots demonstrating the higher degree of scar transmurality on MR imaging (*A*) and the lower degree of inflammation quantified by cardiac MV (*B*) and cardiac MA (*C*) within myocardial segments show the presence of abnormal electrograms compared with those without. (*From* Muser D, Santangeli P, Liang JJ, et al. Characterization of the electroanatomic substrate in cardiac sarcoidosis: correlation with imaging findings of scar and inflammation. JACC Clin Electrophysiol 2018;4:297; with permission.)

segments) (**Fig. 3**).[4] The above data suggest that critical sites for the reentrant VT circuits are strongly associated with presence of scar even in patients with active disease and are located in areas with higher scar transmurality and less evidence of inflammation stressing the central role of fibrosis in the genesis of VAs. In the same series, the authors also found that areas with unipolar voltage abnormalities on electroanatomic voltage mapping correlated with the presence of active inflammation without a significant amount of scar (higher MV and MA and lower degree of scar transmurality in low unipolar voltage areas) representing optimal targets for EMB, thus improving its sensitivity and specificity, which is typically limited by the patchy distribution of the disease and the

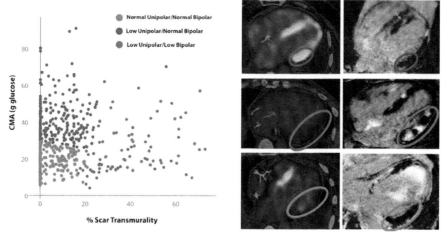

Fig. 3. Correlation among presence of scar, inflammation, and electroanatomic findings in patients with CS undergoing VT ablation. Scatter plot representing the distribution of myocardial segments according to imaging and EAM findings. Segments with both normal unipolar and bipolar voltage (*green dots*) represent the "healthy myocardium" without either scar or inflammation. Segments with low unipolar voltage but normal bipolar voltage (*orange dots*) represent sites of "active disease" with absence/few scar (green *arrows*) and presence of active inflammation (red *arrow*) in which no or only few abnormal electrograms (EGMs) are recorded. Those sites represent potential good targets for EMB. Segments with both low unipolar and bipolar voltage (*blue dots*) represent sites of "advanced disease" with high scar transmurality and no/few inflammatory activity. In such sites, abnormal EGMs are frequently recorded representing potential good targets for substrate modification. CMA, cardiac metabolic activity. (*Adapted from* Muser D, Santangeli P, Liang JJ, et al. Characterization of the electroanatomic substrate in cardiac sarcoidosis: correlation with imaging findings of scar and inflammation. JACC Clin Electrophysiol 2018;4:298; with permission.)

presence of areas with dense scar (nonspecific finding on histology) (see **Fig. 3**).[4] Detection of active inflammation and monitoring its response to immunosuppressive therapy in patients with VAs related to CS have also a significant prognostic impact. The authors initially reported how baseline PET is strongly related to long-term procedural outcomes with a 4-fold increase risk of VT recurrence for those patients with abnormal ^{18}F-FDG uptake and an adjunctive 2-fold increased risk for those with lack of PET improvement after immunosuppressive therapy.[7] Those findings were subsequently confirmed with a more accurate quantitative approach showing how lack of PET improvement (defined by decrease in MA of at least 25%) after initiation of immunosuppressive treatment was associated with a 20-fold higher risk of major adverse cardiac events at follow-up. Moreover, a significant inverse relationship was observed between changes

in MA and changes in left ventricular ejection fraction over follow-up (**Fig. 4**).[6] Similar findings have been reported with the same quantitative approach by Lee and colleagues[17] in a series of 16 patients with CS who underwent serial ^{18}F-FDG-PET during immunosuppressive treatment. To further confirm the pivotal role of inflammation in disease progression, the authors have reported how in patients undergoing a second ablation procedure after a first attempt of CA due to recurrent VT, a significant scar progression was present only in patients with persistent inflammatory activity detected by FDG-PET (**Fig. 5**).[4]

Chagas disease (CD) is a protozoan infection caused by *Trypanosoma cruzi that* can affect many different organs. Cardiac involvement is one of the most frequent manifestations involving approximately one-third of the cases, and it is characterized by conduction system abnormalities, heart failure, and VAs.[18] Progressive cardiac fibrosis related to

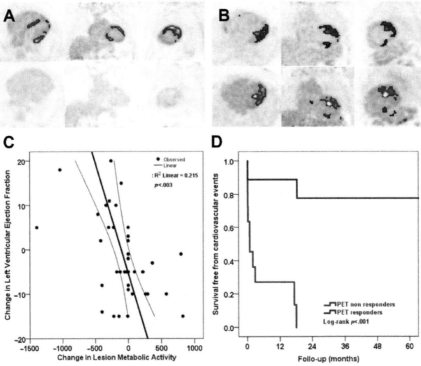

Fig. 4. Correlation between [18]FDG-PET evaluation of treatment response and major adverse cardiac events in patients with CS. (*A*) PET scan in a patient with CS involving the midbasal septum, midbasal anterior, and basal inferior wall of the left ventricle (*A, top row*) that demonstrates complete normalization after 6 months of immunosuppressive therapy (*B, bottom row*). (*B*) Patient with CS involving the lateral and anterior wall of the left ventricle as well as the anterolateral papillary muscle at baseline (*B, top row*) and persistent inflammation of the same areas regardless of 6 months of immunosuppressive treatment (*B, bottom row*). (*C*) Correlation between changes in lesion MA and changes in left ventricular ejection fraction in patients undergoing immunosuppressive treatment of CS and recurrent VT. (*D*) Kaplan-Meier survival curve shows survival free from cardiovascular events according to metabolic response in patients with CS and recurrent VT. (*Adapted from* Muser D, Santangeli P, Castro SA, et al. Prognostic role of serial quantitative evaluation of 18F-fluorodeoxyglucose uptake by PET/CT in patients with cardiac sarcoidosis presenting with ventricular tachycardia. Eur J Nucl Med Mol Imaging. 2018;45(8):1400–1401.; with permission.)

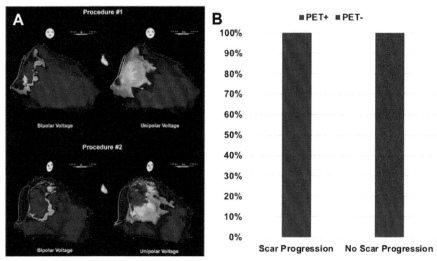

Fig. 5. Correlation between persistent myocardial inflammation and scar progression in patients with CS. (*A*) Endocardial voltage maps of a patient with persistent myocardial inflammation on FDG-PET and evidence of scar progression between 2 consecutive VT CA procedures performed within 3 months. (*B*) Bar chart shows the prevalence of persistent inflammation on FDG-PET among 10 patients with CS who underwent a second ablation procedure after a first attempt of CA due to recurrent VT presenting with (*left bar*) or without (*right bar*) scar progression.

ongoing cardiac inflammation may play a central role in the development of Chagasic cardiomyopathy. Shapiro and colleagues[19] have described 2 cases of CD referred for CA of recurrent VT storm resistant to antiarrhythmic medications who underwent an ^{18}F-FDG-PET before the procedure, finding evidence of active inflammation even in advanced stages of the disease, which may contribute to clinical VT potentially increasing the risk of recurrence after CA in this group of patients.

POTENTIAL PITFALLS OF ^{18}F-FLUORODEOXYGLUCOSE-PET/ COMPUTED TOMOGRAPHY IMAGING FOR DETECTION OF MYOCARDIAL INFLAMMATION

The assumption behind the application of ^{18}F-FDG-PET for the detection of myocardial inflammation is the preferential accumulation of ^{18}F-FDG within inflamed tissue compared with healthy myocardium. Unfortunately, the primary source of cardiac myocytes metabolism is represented by glucose.[20] In this regard, suppression of physiologic myocardial uptake of ^{18}F-FDG is of fundamental importance in order to avoid false positive results and identify areas of true pathologic involvement. Among methods developed to achieve adequate suppression of physiologic ^{18}F-FDG uptake, prolonged fasting ($\geq$18 hours) preceded by a diet of high fat and low carbohydrates is the most commonly used thanks to its capability to force the cardiomyocytes metabolism from a predominant glucose to a

predominant free fatty acid one. Unfortunately, because of the high variability of cardiac ^{18}F-FDG uptake even with prolonged fasting, ^{18}F-FDG-PET specificity remains suboptimal with a substantial risk of false positive results and up to 30% of inconclusive scans.[21] To limit the risk of overestimation of the incidence of abnormal ^{18}F-FDG-PET findings, diffuse homogeneous ^{18}F-FDG uptake is usually considered a result of inadequate suppression, whereas focal or focal on diffuse uptake patterns are usually considered significant. However, to further complicate the interpretation of ^{18}F-FDG-PET results, selective uptake of ^{18}F-FDG in the inferolateral wall even in presence of a complete suppression of the remaining myocardium has been reported as a normal physiologic pattern.[22,23] In this regard, the comparison between ^{18}F-FDG-PET finding and other imaging modalities such CMR with T2-weighted imaging to detect myocardial edema and LGE imaging to detect necrosis/fibrosis may improve the specificity of ^{18}F-FDG-PET findings.[24] Other common sources of false results are represented by misalignment of CT with ^{18}F-FDG-PET scans due to patient movement or abnormal ^{18}F-FDG uptake surrounding pacemaker or implantable cardioverter-defibrillator leads.[25,26]

COMPARISON WITH OTHER IMAGING MODALITIES

A multimodality approach in patients with suspected myocardial inflammation as a source of VAs is usually necessary to increase either diagnostic sensitivity or specificity. In this regard, CMR represents the imaging modality of choice due to its capability of tissue characterization. Discordant findings between CMR and ^{18}F-FDG-PET have been reported in up to 40% of patients with VAs of unexplained origin.[1,11] Similar findings have been described in patients with CS. Ohira and colleagues[16] reported 21 consecutive patients with diagnosis of CS who underwent both ^{18}F-FDG/PET and CMR and found 7 (33%) patients with evidence of abnormal ^{18}F-FDG uptake but no evidence of LGE on MR imaging. Moreover, among 8 (38%) patients with both positive PET and CMR, in 7/8 cases there was imperfect overlap between segments with abnormal FDG-uptake and LGE, and in one patient, the localization of abnormal FDG-uptake was not consistent at all with the distribution of LGE. Vita and colleagues[24] have systematically analyzed the complementary value of CMR imaging and ^{18}F-FDG-PET among 107 patients referred for evaluation of CS. Overall, they reported the presence of LGE in 85% of the patients (66% of them having also evidence of abnormal ^{18}F-FDG uptake) and evidence of abnormal ^{18}F-FDG uptake in 63% of them with a concordance between LGE and ^{18}F-FDG in 76% of the cases. Of note, the combination of PET information to CMR determined a reclassification to having a higher or lower likelihood of CS in about 45% of the examined cases. In this study, half of the patients without evidence of LGE on CMR had evidence of abnormal ^{18}F-FDG uptake; however, only 50% of them were ultimately categorized as having a high probability of CS on the final diagnosis. Similarly, Soussan and colleagues[27] evaluated 35 patients with suspected CS by CMR and PET and found 3 individuals with positive ^{18}F-FDG who had negative LGE with none of them matching the Japanese Ministry of Health, Labour, and Welfare criteria. The discordant findings on ^{18}F-FDG and MR imaging may be explained by the capacity of each of the 2 modalities to detect different pathologic attributes of the same disease. Focal ^{18}F-FDG uptake reflects the presence of inflammation due to its capacity to accumulate in cells with augmented glucose uptake.[28] On the other hand, high signal on T2-weighted imaging and LGE represents edema and/or increased extracellular space.[29] In most of the cases, there is a large overlap between abnormal ^{18}F-FDG uptake visible on PET and areas of LGE visible on CMR, but the presence of focal ^{18}F-FDG uptake in the absence of CMR alterations may be explained by inflammation-related microvascular obstruction, whereas on the counterpart sites showing LGE without any evidence of ^{18}F-FDG uptake, represents areas of advanced disease with no residual viability (see **Figs. 2** and

3). Although the absence of LGE on CMR can rule out disease in most patients, ^{18}F-FDG-PET provides a better assessment of the presence and extent of myocardial inflammation and should always be performed especially in cases of equivocal or negative CMR.[24] Recently, the development of new radiotracers, which do not physiologically accumulate within healthy myocardium, such as Gallium-68 (^{68}Ga) DOTATAE, may potentially overcome ^{18}F-FDG limitations. ^{68}Ga-DOTATAE was initially developed to assess neuroendocrine tumors because it targets somatostatin receptors; however, it subsequently demonstrated to target also activated macrophages as they express somatostatin receptors.[30] Considering the absence of such receptors on normal myocardial cells, ^{68}Ga-DOTATAE could possibly represent a selective marker of myocardial inflammation, thus reducing the incidence of false positive scans and the need for laborious patent preparation.[31,32]

OTHER APPLICATIONS OF PET IMAGING

Various other PET modalities can be used to identify different pathophysiologic aspects of the arrhythmic substrate of VAs and guide CA. Depending on the pathway of the specific tracer used, PET imaging can identify areas of abnormal myocardial perfusion, scar metabolism, and sympathetic innervation. Single-photon emission computed tomography (SPECT) is a well-established technique to identify myocardial scar; however, PET provides advantages over SPECT, including higher spatial resolution and the ability of absolute quantification of myocardial blood flow.[33] In between PET tracers, ^{15}O-water is considered the gold standard because it is freely diffusible and metabolically inert, allowing assessment of even subtle perfusion abnormalities. In a recent study including 30 patients with ischemic cardiomyopathy, impaired perfusion quantified by ^{15}O-water PET was significantly related with VT inducibility on electrophysiological study.[34] Myocardial viability is commonly assessed with ^{18}F-FDG-PET because ^{18}F-FDG uptake is preserved in viable myocardium, whereas reduced uptake indicates nonviable scar tissue. Scar tissue is generally defined by an ^{18}F-FDG uptake $\leq$50% of normalized maximum uptake.[35] A good correlation between [18]F-FDG-PET–based scar and voltage mapping has been reported. In their initial experience in 14 patients treated with CA for drug-refractory VT, Dickfeld and colleagues[36] demonstrated that PET defined scar ($\leq$50% MA) had a sensitivity of 89% and a specificity of 93% in predicting areas of abnormal voltage. In another study including 10 patients who underwent ^{18}F-FDG-PET before CA of

VT, areas of low voltage had significantly lower levels of MA compared with areas of normal voltage (40% vs 89%, respectively) with a metabolic threshold of 46% demonstrating the best discriminatory power between areas of voltage abnormality and healthy myocardium.[37] In a study integrating perfusion imaging with [82]Rb PET and metabolism with ^{18}F-FDG-PET, the metabolic scar (defined as <50% uptake) appeared to be best correlated by a voltage threshold of 0.9 mV compared with the typical 1.5 mV one. Interestingly, in this study, all the effective ablation sites were located within the PET defined scar.[38] Another important field of application of PET imaging involves the study of cardiac sympathetic innervation. Sympathetic hyperactivity plays a central role in the genesis and maintenance of VAs, and there is growing evidence that its modulation by cardiac deafferentation may be an effective treatment strategy in patients presenting with refractory VAs.[39,40] In this regard, nuclear imaging represents a valuable tool to assess cardiac sympathetic innervation. The most commonly used radiotracers are ^{123}I-meta-iodobenzylguanidine (^{123}I-mIBG) for SPECT and ^{11}C-HED for PET; both are analogues of norepinephrine that constitute the presynaptic neuromodulator of sympathetic terminations and have high affinity for presynaptic norepinephrine reuptake transporters, thus visualizing presynaptic sympathetic terminations.[41] ^{123}I-mIBG-SPECT has been shown to predict occurrence of ICD shocks in patients with heart failure.[42] Areas of abnormal cardiac sympathetic innervation may also represent good targets for CA of VT. In a study involving 15 patients with ischemic cardiomyopathy undergoing VT CA, and preprocedural ^{123}I-mIBG-SPECT, the totality of effective ablation sites were located within areas of abnormal innervation, whereas only 64% of them were within areas of low voltage defined by classical thresholds.[43] A greater VT inducibility on electrophysiological study was also demonstrated in patients with ischemic cardiomyopathy and larger areas of denervation determined by ^{123}I-mIBG-SPECT.[44] Some preliminary data in animal models of healed myocardial infarction have shown how the extent of viable but denervated myocardium quantified by ^{11}C-epinephrine and ^{13}N-ammonia PET was correlated not only with VT inducibility on electrophysiological testing but also with the site of origin of induced VTs and the extent of voltage abnormality on electroanatomic mapping.[45]

SUMMARY

PET imaging has an increasing role in the field of cardiac electrophysiology, helping in diagnosis, risk stratification, and management of patients with complex VAs. Depending on the particular radiotracer used, PET imaging can assess different pathophysiologic aspects of the arrhythmogenic substrate by evaluating cardiac perfusion, myocardial inflammation, viability, and sympathetic innervation. The integration of PET imaging with electroanatomic mapping systems could also potentially improve VT ablation outcomes by identifying critical sites for VT.

REFERENCES

1. Tung R, Bauer B, Schelbert H, et al. Incidence of abnormal positron emission tomography in patients with unexplained cardiomyopathy and ventricular arrhythmias: the potential role of occult inflammation in arrhythmogenesis. Heart Rhythm 2015;12:2488–98.
2. Nucifora G, Muser D, Masci PG, et al. Prevalence and prognostic value of concealed structural abnormalities in patients with apparently idiopathic ventricular arrhythmias of left versus right ventricular origin a magnetic resonance imaging study. Circ Arrhythm Electrophysiol 2014;7:456–62.
3. Lazzerini PE, Capecchi PL, Laghi-Pasini F. Systemic inflammation and arrhythmic risk: lessons from rheumatoid arthritis. Eur Heart J 2017;38(22):1717–27.
4. Muser D, Santangeli P, Liang JJ, et al. Characterization of the electroanatomic substrate in cardiac sarcoidosis: correlation with imaging findings of scar and inflammation. JACC Clin Electrophysiol 2018;4:291–303.
5. Bertini M, Schalij MJ, Bax JJ, et al. Emerging role of multimodality imaging to evaluate patients at risk for sudden cardiac death. Circ Cardiovasc Imaging 2012;5:525–35.
6. Muser D, Santangeli P, Castro SA, et al. Prognostic role of serial quantitative evaluation of ^{18}F-fluorodeoxyglucose uptake by PET/CT in patients with cardiac sarcoidosis presenting with ventricular tachycardia. Eur J Nucl Med Mol Imaging 2018; 45(8):1394–404.
7. Muser D, Santangeli P, Pathak RK, et al. Long-term outcomes of catheter ablation of ventricular tachycardia in patients with cardiac sarcoidosis. Circ Arrhythm Electrophysiol 2016;9:e004333.
8. Stevenson WG, Khan H, Sager P, et al. Identification of reentry circuit sites during catheter mapping and radiofrequency ablation of ventricular tachycardia late after myocardial infarction. Circulation 1993;88:1647–70.
9. Budzianowski JK, Korybalska K, Bręborowicz A. The role of inflammation in cardiac arrhythmias pathophysiology. J Med Sci 2016;85:197–204.
10. Klein RM, Vester EG, Brehm MU, et al. [Inflammation of the myocardium as an arrhythmia trigger]. Z Kardiol 2000;89(Suppl 3):24–35.

11. Lakkireddy D, Yarlagadda B, Turagam M, et al. B-LBCT02-02. Myocarditis is an underrecognized etiology of symptomatic premature ventricular contractions - insights from the myocarditis and ventricular arrhythmia (MAVERIC) registry. Heart Rhythm 2018;15:942–5.

12. Birnie DH, Nery PB, Ha AC, et al. Cardiac sarcoidosis. J Am Coll Cardiol 2016;68:411–21.

13. Kumar S, Barbhaiya C, Nagashima K, et al. Ventricular tachycardia in cardiac sarcoidosis characterization of ventricular substrate and outcomes of catheter ablation. Circ Arrhythm Electrophysiol 2015;8:87–93.

14. Segawa M, Fukuda K, Nakano M, et al. Time course and factors correlating with ventricular tachyarrhythmias after introduction of steroid therapy in cardiac sarcoidosis. Circ Arrhythm Electrophysiol 2016;9: e003353.

15. Patel MR, Cawley PJ, Heitner JF, et al. Detection of myocardial damage in patients with sarcoidosis. Circulation 2009;120:1969–77.

16. Ohira H, Tsujino I, Ishimaru S, et al. Myocardial imaging with 18F-fluoro-2-deoxyglucose positron emission tomography and magnetic resonance imaging in sarcoidosis. Eur J Nucl Med Mol Imaging 2007;35:933–41.

17. Lee P-I, Cheng G, Alavi A. The role of serial FDG PET for assessing therapeutic response in patients with cardiac sarcoidosis. J Nucl Cardiol 2017; 24(1):19–28.

18. Bestetti RB, Muccillo G. Clinical course of Chagas' heart disease: a comparison with dilated cardiomyopathy. Int J Cardiol 1997;60:187–93.

19. Shapiro H, Meymandi S, Shivkumar K, et al. Cardiac inflammation and ventricular tachycardia in Chagas disease. Heartrhythm Case Rep 2017;3:392–5.

20. Camici P, Ferrannini E, Opie LH. Myocardial metabolism in ischemic heart disease: basic principles and application to imaging by positron emission tomography. Prog Cardiovasc Dis 1989;32:217–38.

21. Manabe O, Yoshinaga K, Ohira H, et al. The effects of 18-h fasting with low-carbohydrate diet preparation on suppressed physiological myocardial 18F-fluorodeoxyglucose (FDG) uptake and possible minimal effects of unfractionated heparin use in patients with suspected cardiac involvement sarcoidosis. J Nucl Cardiol 2016;23:244–52.

22. Choi Y, Brunken RC, Hawkins RA, et al. Factors affecting myocardial 2-[F-18]fluoro-2-deoxy-D-glucose uptake in positron emission tomography studies of normal humans. Eur J Nucl Med 1993; 20:308–18.

23. Iozzo P, Chareonthaitawee P, Di Terlizzi M, et al. Regional myocardial blood flow and glucose utilization during fasting and physiological hyperinsulinemia in humans. Am J Physiol Endocrinol Metab 2002;282:E1163–71.

24. Vita T, Okada DR, Veillet-Chowdhury M, et al. Complementary value of cardiac magnetic resonance imaging and positron emission tomography/computed tomography in the assessment of cardiac sarcoidosis. Circ Cardiovasc Imaging 2018;11(1): e007030.

25. Dilsizian V, Bacharach SL, Beanlands RS, et al. ASNC imaging guidelines/SNMMI procedure standard for positron emission tomography (PET) nuclear cardiology procedures. J Nucl Cardiol 2016; 23:1187–226.

26. DiFilippo FP, Brunken RC. Do implanted pacemaker leads and ICD leads cause metal-related artifact in cardiac PET/CT? J Nucl Med 2005;46:436–43.

27. Soussan M, Brillet P-Y, Nunes H, et al. Clinical value of a high-fat and low-carbohydrate diet before FDG-PET/CT for evaluation of patients with suspected cardiac sarcoidosis. J Nucl Cardiol 2013;20:120–7.

28. Kubota R, Yamada S, Kubota K, et al. Intratumoral distribution of fluorine-18-fluorodeoxyglucose in vivo: high accumulation in macrophages and granulation tissues studied by microautoradiography. J Nucl Med 1992;33:1972–80.

29. Selvanayagam J, Nucifora GG. Early and late gadolinium enhancement. The EACVI textbook of cardiovascular magnetic resonance. Oxford (NY): Oxford University Press; 2018.

30. Mojtahedi A, Thamake S, Tworowska I, et al. The value of (68)Ga-DOTATATE PET/CT in diagnosis and management of neuroendocrine tumors compared to current FDA approved imaging modalities: a review of literature. Am J Nucl Med Mol Imaging 2014;4:426–34.

31. Gormsen LC, Haraldsen A, Kramer S, et al. A dual tracer (68)Ga-DOTANOC PET/CT and (18)F-FDG PET/CT pilot study for detection of cardiac sarcoidosis. EJNMMI Res 2016;6:52.

32. Lapa C, Reiter T, Kircher M, et al. Somatostatin receptor based PET/CT in patients with the suspicion of cardiac sarcoidosis: an initial comparison to cardiac MRI. Oncotarget 2016;7:77807–14.

33. Knaapen P, de Haan S, Hoekstra OS, et al. Cardiac PET-CT: advanced hybrid imaging for the detection of coronary artery disease. Neth Heart J 2010;18:90–8.

34. Rijnierse MT, de Haan S, Harms HJ, et al. Impaired hyperemic myocardial blood flow is associated with inducibility of ventricular arrhythmia in ischemic cardiomyopathy. Circ Cardiovasc Imaging 2014;7: 20–30.

35. Schinkel AFL, Poldermans D, Elhendy A, et al. Assessment of myocardial viability in patients with heart failure. J Nucl Med 2007;48:1135–46.

36. Dickfeld T, Lei P, Dilsizian V, et al. Integration of three-dimensional scar maps for ventricular tachycardia ablation with positron emission tomography-computed tomography. JACC Cardiovasc Imaging 2008;1:73–82.

37. Tian J, Smith MF, Chinnadurai P, et al. Clinical application of PET/CT fusion imaging for three-dimensional myocardial scar and left ventricular anatomy during ventricular tachycardia ablation. J Cardiovasc Electrophysiol 2009;20:567–604.

38. Fahmy TS, Wazni OM, Jaber WA, et al. Integration of positron emission tomography/computed tomography with electroanatomical mapping: a novel approach for ablation of scar-related ventricular tachycardia. Heart Rhythm 2008;5:1538–45.

39. Vaseghi M, Gima J, Kanaan C, et al. Cardiac sympathetic denervation in patients with refractory ventricular arrhythmias or electrical storm: intermediate and long-term follow-up. Heart Rhythm 2014;11:360–6.

40. Vaseghi M, Barwad P, Malavassi Corrales FJ, et al. Cardiac sympathetic denervation for refractory ventricular arrhythmias. J Am Coll Cardiol 2017;69:3070–80.

41. Thackeray JT, Bengel FM. Assessment of cardiac autonomic neuronal function using PET imaging. J Nucl Cardiol 2013;20:150–65.

42. Boogers MJ, Borleffs CJW, Henneman MM, et al. Cardiac sympathetic denervation assessed with 123-iodine metaiodobenzylguanidine imaging predicts ventricular arrhythmias in implantable cardioverter-defibrillator patients. J Am Coll Cardiol 2010;55:2769–77.

43. Klein T, Abdulghani M, Smith M, et al. Three-dimensional 123I-meta-iodobenzylguanidine cardiac innervation maps to assess substrate and successful ablation sites for ventricular tachycardia: feasibility study for a novel paradigm of innervation imaging. Circ Arrhythm Electrophysiol 2015;8:583–91.

44. Bax JJ, Kraft O, Buxton AE, et al. 123 I-mIBG scintigraphy to predict inducibility of ventricular arrhythmias on cardiac electrophysiology testing: a prospective multicenter pilot study. Circ Cardiovasc Imaging 2008;1:131–40.

45. Sasano T, Abraham MR, Chang K-C, et al. Abnormal sympathetic innervation of viable myocardium and the substrate of ventricular tachycardia after myocardial infarction. J Am Coll Cardiol 2008;51:2266–75.

Current and Future Cardiovascular PET Radiopharmaceuticals

Rami Al-Haddad, Uzair S. Ismailani,
Benjamin H. Rotstein, PhD*

KEYWORDS

- Cardiovascular diseases • Positron emission tomography imaging • Radiotracers
- Myocardial blood flow • Atherosclerosis • Fatty acid metabolism
- Cardiac autonomic nervous system

KEY POINTS

- Molecular imaging of cardiovascular diseases is an established approach to diagnose conditions and manage patient care.
- PET is an evolving noninvasive imaging technique that can be used to better understand the mechanisms and pathologies of cardiovascular diseases.
- PET relies on sensitive and selective radiopharmaceuticals.
- Future PET radiotracers are being developed to accurately quantify markers of pathology in cardiovascular disease with greater disease specificity.

INTRODUCTION

Despite meaningful advances in the treatment and prevention of cardiovascular diseases (CVD), these remains the primary cause of mortality and morbidity worldwide, with stroke and ischemic heart disease causing more than 15 million deaths per year globally.[1,2] CVD includes various heart- and vessel-related conditions of different etiologies.[3] Coronary artery disease (CAD) affects any vessel supplying blood to the heart and is characterized by defects in blood flow often caused by atherosclerosis.[4] An increasing appreciation of the complex roles of inflammation, calcification, and tissue remodeling in CAD and valvular CVD are leading to a better understanding and classification of these conditions. Congestive heart failure and associated complications such as ventricular arrhythmias can result from various underlying causes, including autonomic nervous system failure, ischemia, and hypoxia.[5]

Mechanisms and therapeutic strategies directed toward CVD have naturally been the subject of investigation for many years, including advances in sensitive and specific diagnostic methods.[6] The year 1927 marks the birth of diagnostic nuclear medicine, when Blumgart and Weiss[7] measured circulation time from one arm to the other in volunteers and patients without CVD using bismuth-214 (^{214}Bi; half-life $t_{1/2} = 26.8$ minutes). Almost 2 decades later, Prinzmetal and colleagues[8] used a Geiger-Müller tube to measure the blood transit time between the left and right ventricles by generating a radiocardiogram after a bolus injection of sodium-24. Since these seminal studies, myriad isotopes

Disclosure Statement: The authors have no disclosures.
Financial support for this work was provided by the University of Ottawa Heart Institute and the Ontario Ministry of Research and Innovation Early Researcher Award ER17-13-119.
Department of Biochemistry, Microbiology and Immunology, University of Ottawa, University of Ottawa Heart Institute, 40 Ruskin Street, Ottawa, Ontario K1Y 4E9, Canada
* Corresponding author. H-5219, 40 Ruskin Street, Ottawa, Ontario K1Y 4W7, Canada.
E-mail address: benjamin.rotstein@uottawa.ca

PET Clin 14 (2019) 293–305
https://doi.org/10.1016/j.cpet.2018.12.010

and tracers have been tested preclinically and clinically to eventually develop the currently available and future imaging radiopharmaceuticals.

Various cardiovascular imaging modalities are now at clinicians' disposal to diagnose or assess the progression of CVDs in patients.[9] These include echocardiography, radiographs, computed tomography, magnetic resonance imaging, planar scintigraphy, single-photon emission computed tomography (SPECT), and positron emission tomography (PET).[9] This review article focuses on PET radiotracers available for CVD and their clinical applications. PET radiopharmaceuticals are labeled with positron-emitting isotopes. These agents produce a pair of antiparallel 511 keV photons following decay and a subsequent positronium annihilation event.[10] PET detectors are equipped with coincident γ-photon detectors to record decays with high sensitivity. Dynamic and quantifiable images can then be reconstructed with moderate spatial and temporal resolution.[10] Well-characterized and selective radiopharmaceuticals are then truly the strength of PET, because they enable unparalleled biochemical resolution to probe targets and mechanisms of CVD under various imaging conditions.[4] These tracers, along with ongoing advances in PET technology point toward better tools for the diagnosis and assessment of CVD.

PET ISOTOPES FOR CARDIOVASCULAR DISEASE IMAGING

There are several considerations for selection of a PET isotope for a clinical CVD radiopharmaceutical. The physical half-life must be suitable for the kinetics of tracer distribution and any targeted biochemical processes, and may place constraints on chemical synthesis, imaging protocols such as exercise for stress testing, or dosimetry. An on-site cyclotron is required for short-lived radioisotopes not available from generators. An ideal PET isotope would decay entirely through positron (β^+) emission. Image resolution is also affected by β^+ energy, as a function of its range in water. Ultimately, although PET isotopes with a variety of physical properties and production methods are available, the selection of a nuclide often depends on molecular structures and synthetic feasibility.[11,12]

Carbon-11 (^{11}C)

- $t_{1/2}$ = 20.34 minutes
- 99.8% β^+, E_{mean} = 0.386   MeV, $R_{mean} \cdot H_2O$ = 1.2 mm
- Cyclotron-produced in nitrogen gas: $^{14}N(p,\alpha)^{11}C$
- [^{11}C]CO_2 or [^{11}C]CH_4 precursors, complex synthesis possible

Nitrogen-13 (^{13}N)

- $t_{1/2}$ = 9.96 minutes
- 99.8% β^+, E_{mean} = 0.492   MeV, $R_{mean} \cdot H_2O$ = 1.2 mm
- Cyclotron-produced in water: $^{16}O(p,\alpha)^{13}N$
- [^{13}N]NH_3 or [^{13}N]NO_3^- precursors, complex synthesis uncommon

Oxygen-15 (^{15}O)

- $t_{1/2}$ = 2.04 minutes
- 99.9% β^+, E_{mean} = 0.735   MeV, $R_{mean} \cdot H_2O$ = 1.2 mm
- Cyclotron-produced in nitrogen gas: $^{14}N(d,n)^{15}O$ or $^{15}N(p,n)^{15}O$
- [^{15}O]O_2 is most common precursor, single-step synthesis possible

Fluorine-18 (^{18}F)

- $t_{1/2}$ = 109.7 minutes
- 96.9% β^+, E_{mean} = 0.250   MeV, $R_{mean} \cdot H_2O$ = 1.2 mm
- Cyclotron-produced in enriched water: $^{18}O(p,n)^{18}F$
- [^{18}F]fluoride most common precursor, complex synthesis possible

Copper-64 (^{64}Cu)

- $t_{1/2}$ = 12.7 h
- 17.5% β^+, E_{mean} = 0.278   MeV, $R_{mean} \cdot H_2O$ = 1.2 mm
- Cyclotron-produced: $^{64}Ni(p,n)^{64}Cu$
- Chelation chemistry

Gallium-68 (^{68}Ga)

- $t_{1/2}$ = 67.8 minutes
- 88.9% β^+, E_{mean} = 0.836   MeV, $R_{mean} \cdot H_2O$ = 1.2 mm
- Generator produced from germanium-68
- Chelation chemistry

Rubidium-82 (^{82}Rb)

- $t_{1/2}$ = 1.25 minutes
- 94.9% β^+, E_{mean} = 1.535   MeV, $R_{mean} \cdot H_2O$ = 1.2 mm
- Generator produced from strontium-82
- Used as eluted

PET RADIOTRACERS USED FOR CARDIOVASCULAR DISEASE IMAGING

Detection and Monitoring of Stenosis Through Cardiac PET Imaging: Coronary Artery Disease Definition and Symptoms

CAD is characterized by the narrowing of blood vessels, affecting normal blood flow. Symptoms range from shortness of breath to chest pain and, in some cases, may lead to acute events such as myocardial infarction and ischemia. Using PET, it has been shown that impaired myocardial blood flow (MBF) is a hallmark of an increased relative risk of progression of heart failure and death.[13] PET imaging can be used to provide noninvasive evaluation of coronary arterial function by assessing regional MBF within the left ventricle. For MBF, PET images are acquired when patients are at rest and under stress.[14] The images can then be reconstructed and analyzed to provide left ventricular MBF values (in milliliters per minute per gram), as well as the myocardial flow reserve, which is the ratio of MBF during stress and at rest.[15] Although many studies highlight the use of PET in CAD, it is believed that PET is still underused in clinical diagnosis of heart and vascular abnormalities.[16]

[13N]Ammonia

[13N]Ammonia (**Fig. 1**) was first produced by Curie and Joliot in 1934 and was found to have a half-life of approximately 10 minutes and to decay by β^+ emission, producing [13C].[17] This tracer is taken up as ammonia in the heart by free diffusion across the cell membranes and equilibrates with the ammonium ion.[18] It becomes trapped inside the cell after it is converted to [13N]glutamine by glutamine synthase. The metabolic fate of [13N]ammonia was assessed, and it was found that the most predominant metabolite was [13N]urea, followed by neutral amino acids such as [13N]glutamine and [13N]asparagine.[19] The time course of the tracer parent fraction in plasma is species dependent, and can impact image interpretation, although metabolism is relatively slower in humans.[20] In comparison with microspheres, the myocardial extraction coefficient of [13N]ammonia is nonlinear at higher flow rates.[21] Although single-photon emission computed tomography has been widely used as a diagnostic tool for CVD, the use of [13N]ammonia in PET offers a greater diagnostic capacity with remarkable accuracy.[22] A linear relationship was established between MBF and tracer concentration, indicating the usefulness of [13N]ammonia as an imaging agent for MBF.

[15O]Water

This tracer is taken up through passive diffusion across cell membranes.[23] Out of all perfusion tracers, it is shown that only [15O]water (see **Fig. 1**) displays a linear relationship between MBF and myocardial extraction, allowing MBF quantification over a wide range of values.[24] Analytical approaches to PET images obtained using [15O]water may be improved by correction of baseline MBF values using an index of myocardial oxygen consumption and other factors, including the gender, age, and body mass.[25] Still, [15O]water remains the most accurate PET radiotracer for MBF over a wide range of values.[26]

[18F]Flurpiridaz

[18F]Flurpiridaz (see **Fig. 1**) is an inhibitor of the mitochondrial complex-1 of the electron transport chain and a promising perfusion PET tracer, currently in phase III clinical trials. In biodistribution studies, [18F]flurpiridaz shows high uptake in the heart and its high myocardial extraction fraction is useful in quantifying MBF using PET.[27] The long physical half-life of [18F] makes [18F]flurpiridaz a convenient tracer for clinical use, compared with other tracers such as [82Rb] and [13N]ammonia.[28] Clinical trials using [18F]flurpiridaz showed high diagnostic certainty.[29] Furthermore, [18F]flurpiridaz was evaluated to also be superior to commonly used single-photon emission computed tomography imaging tracers.[30] This tracer also demonstrated excellent extraction fractions over a range of physiologic values.[14]

Rubidium-82

Interest in rubidium-82 for imaging emerged in 1954 when Love and colleagues[31] demonstrated that its heart uptake was proportional to blood flow in the coronary arteries. Rubidium is taken up by the myocardium from the blood through a Na^+/K^+-ATPase.[32] [82Rb] uptake has been shown to be unaffected by pharmacologic or metabolic interventions.[33] However, myocardial extraction is even more dependent on flow rates for this tracer than with respect to [13N]ammonia, rendering it insensitive at high flow.[34] The first injection of [82Rb] in humans took place in 1980, where it was shown that the resulting PET images possessed a high diagnostic accuracy for MBF quantification.[35] Since its approval by the US Food and Drug Administration in 1989, [82Rb] has been used extensively with PET and emerged as an essential tool in measuring MBF and coronary

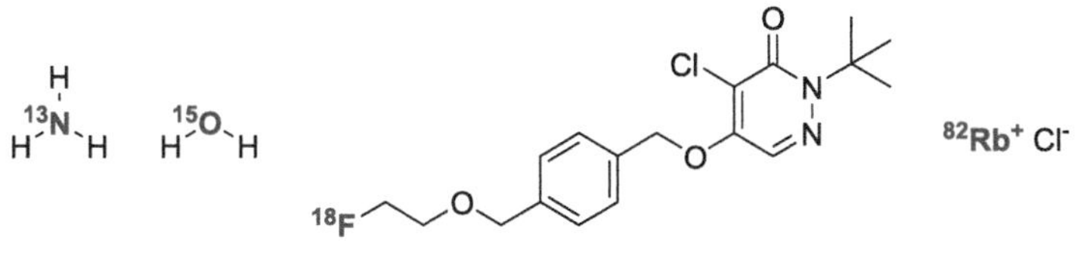

Fig. 1. Structures of [13N]ammonia, [15O]water, [18F]flurpiridaz, and [82Rb]rubidium chloride.

reserve.[36] One major limitation of [82]Rb was the high radiation doses required owing to its short physical half-life. Currently, PET scans using lower [82]Rb activity are being tested to reach an optimal image resolution with the lowest dosimetry possible.[24] Based on a database established previously, it was found that, with camera advancements, [82]Rb PET displays greater accuracy in diagnosing patients with CAD than [^{13}N]ammonia, as well as those with a high risk of CAD incidence.[37] Currently, [82]Rb is regarded as a standard for the imaging of CAD.[24]

[^{18}F](4-Fluorophenyl)triphenylphosphonium cation

Tetraphenylphosphonium has been shown to be a marker of the mitochondrial membrane potential. Mechanistically, it relies on mitochondrial uptake of lipophilic cations.[38] Recently, the tetraphenylphosphonium cation was labeled with ^{18}F to produce [^{18}F]TPP (Fig. 2) for PET imaging of MBF through quantifying myocardial membrane potential.[39,40] It has been established that inhibition of ATP production affected by a decrease in mitochondrial membrane potential is a marker of heart failure.[38] Rodent studies have hinted at the value of measuring the mitochondrial membrane potential in the prognosis of heart failure, because any decrease in this potential will have significant effects on the pathophysiology of the heart. An initial study using swine found an overestimation of myocardial membrane potential owing to nonspecific uptake, rendering this tracer useful for relative but not absolute quantification of MBF.[38]

Radiotracers for the Early Detection of Atherosclerosis Progression and Adverse Effects

Atherosclerosis is a slowly progressive disease leading to many heart- and vessel-related complications. It is characterized by the accumulation of fibrous elements and lipids in the large arteries. Early on, subendothelial accumulations of macrophages filled with cholesterol, known as foam cells, cause the characteristic lesions of atherosclerosis.[41] Fatty streaks alone are not considered to be clinically significant. However, their presence signals the possibility of advanced lesions distinguished by the accumulation of lipid-rich necrotic

debris in addition to smooth muscle cells. These lesions have a fibrous cap that is formed of extracellular matrix and smooth muscle cells, enclosing the lipid-rich necrotic core. Atherosclerotic plaques are subject to an increase in complexity; they are prone to calcification and luminal surface ulceration. Furthermore, small vessels originating from the media of the vessel wall can grow into the fibrous lesions, causing severe hemorrhage.[42] Advanced lesions may cause stenosis and even completely block blood flow. The most significant clinical risk is the acute occlusion of the artery caused by a blood clot or thrombus, leading to a myocardial infarction or stroke. This event is most common after the rupture of a lesion.[41] Numerous markers of atherosclerosis have been identified and are being exploited by different studies to assess the degree of disease progression.[43]

[^{18}F]2-Deoxy-2-fluoro-D-glucose ([^{18}F]FDG)

[^{18}F]FDG (Fig. 3) uptake has been validated as a marker of atherosclerotic plaque inflammation.[44] [^{18}F]FDG is taken up by the cell and phosphorylated by hexokinase, but does not undergo glycolysis. Therefore, the tracer is trapped in the cell and serves as a marker for high metabolic energy consumption.[44] In a recent clinical study, [^{18}F]FDG uptake and CD68 expression in atherosclerotic plaques were found to be correlated.[45] Therefore, [^{18}F]FDG serves as an inflammatory marker and can be useful in assessing atherosclerosis progression. However, [^{18}F]FDG uptake is known to be unspecific, because the tracer binds to inflammatory macrophages among other cell types and shows uptake in organs with high metabolic activity, such as the heart. As a result, myocardial uptake can mask the signal in vascular—especially coronary—plaques. Therefore, markers with greater specificity are needed to identify inflammation in atherosclerotic plaques using PET.[46]

Sodium [^{18}F]fluoride

Calcification of atherosclerotic plaques is another marker for progressive disease and lesion instability. Unlike active microcalcifications, macrocalcifications are associated with stable plaques.[47] These can amplify mechanical stress in the

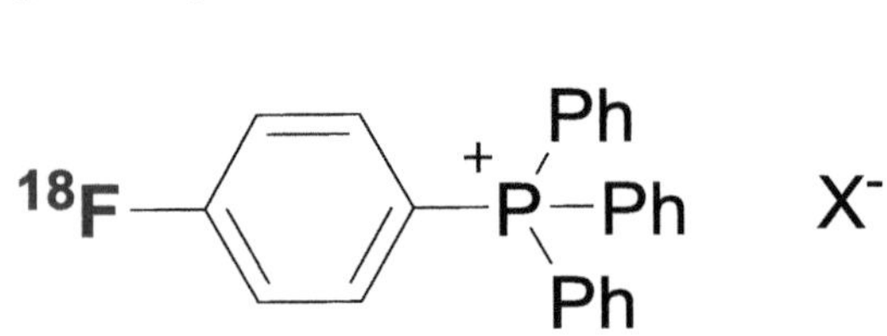

Fig. 2. Structure of [^{18}F]TPP.

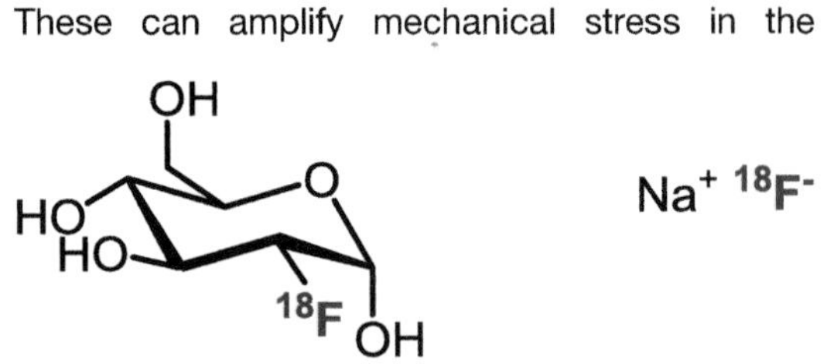

Fig. 3. Structures of [^{18}F]FDG and [^{18}F]NaF.

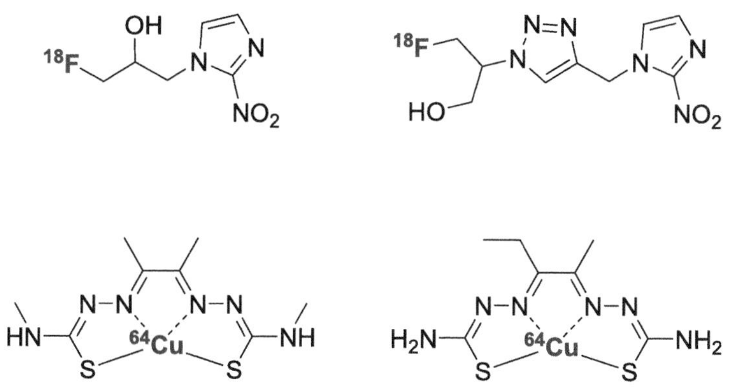

Fig. 4. Structures of [18F]FMISO, [18F]HX4, [64Cu]ATSM, [64Cu]CTS.

atherosclerotic cap by more than 500 kPa, increasing the risk of plaque rupture.[48] [18F]NaF (see **Fig. 3**) is a PET tracer approved by the US Food and Drug Administration. It binds to regions of microcalcification in atherosclerotic plaques.[47] As it binds to hydroxyapatite by replacing its hydroxyl groups, it is considered to be a selective marker of active microcalcification.[49] Recently, a study by Cocker and colleagues[44] showed increased uptake of [18F]NaF with increased hydroxyapatite expression. This finding was also correlated with increased plaque instability.[48] Although calcium has been considered to be a static material, dynamic remodeling of calcific lesions may contribute to plaque instability.[44]

Hypoxia Radiotracers: Nidazoles and Bis(thiosemicarbazones)

Hypoxia is a feature of advanced coronary atherosclerosis and promotes neovascularization and progression of complex plaques.[50] Hypoxia can be molecularly characterized by the presence of hypoxia-inducible factor-1α and is associated with increased lipid accumulation and low-density lipoprotein oxidation.[51] Indeed, mounting evidence from in vitro and in vivo clinical imaging studies suggests that [18F]FDG uptake in atherosclerotic plaques is strongly influenced by hypoxia, as opposed to inflammation.[52,53] The nitroimidazole class of radiotracers is reactive toward single electron species and, in the absence of oxygen, generates radiolabeled alkylating (and therefore residualizing) agents to mark hypoxic cells.[54] This class includes [18F]FMISO (**Fig. 4**), which has been tested in animal models of atherosclerosis[55] and a prospective human study,[52] as well as [18F]HX4 (see **Fig. 4**), which has also advanced for human imaging.[56]

Similar to nitroimidazoles, bis(thiosemicarbazone) organometallic complexes undergo reduction in hypoxic environments, releasing a metal that is trapped intracellularly. The leading radiotracers in this class are [64Cu]ATSM and [64Cu]CTS (see **Fig. 4**), both of which have been studied in preclinical models.[57–59] Studies in perfused rat hearts suggest that [64Cu]CTS has greater sensitivity to low-grade hypoxia compared with other tracers in this class, which could provide clinical advantages.[60]

Translocator Protein Radiotracers: [11C]PK11195 and [18F]GE180

Translocator protein has emerged as a valuable imaging marker for neuroinflammation and the target of numerous radiotracer development programs.[61] These ligands, in particular [11C](R)-PK11195 (**Fig. 5**), have been repurposed for imaging inflammation in atherosclerosis. Although this tracer colocalizes with CD68 inflammation markers by immunohistochemistry,[62,63] it suffers from low specificity and sensitivity in the target tissues.[64,65] A recent study of [18F]GE180 (see **Fig. 5**) tracked increasing levels of translocator protein in the myocardia and brains of mice after coronary artery ligation. Neuroinflammation followed both the infarct and progressive heart failure.[65] These studies chart a path to understanding the molecular signatures of the brain–heart axis in patients suffering from CVD.

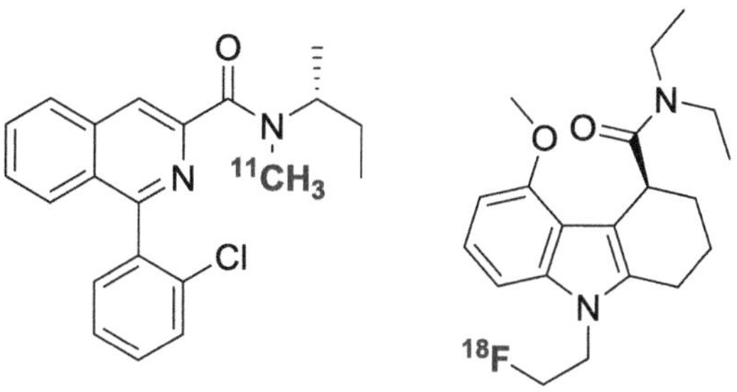

Fig. 5. Structures of [11C](R)-PK11195 and [18F]GE180.

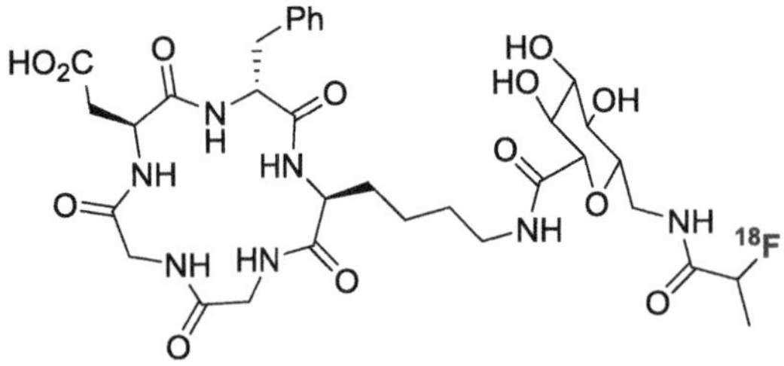

Fig. 6. Structure of [18F]Galacto-RGD.

[18F]Galacto-RGD

[18F]Galacto-RGD (**Fig. 6**) is a PET tracer that binds specifically to $\alpha_v\beta_3$ integrin, which is highly expressed in macrophages and endothelial cells, notably in atherosclerotic plaques.[63] Using autoradiography, it was shown that uptake of [18F]galacto-RGD localizes specifically to atherosclerotic plaques. In addition, PET images and biodistribution data showed a significantly higher uptake in atherosclerotic model mice compared to control mice.[63] Imaging tumors and markers of cell death have emerged as a greater emphasis for [18F]galacto-RGD PET.[66]

[68Ga]DOTATATE

[68Ga]DOTATATE (**Fig. 7**) is a PET ligand that specifically binds to the somatostatin receptor subtype-2 with high affinity.[67] Somatostatin receptor subtype-2 is considered to be a better marker of macrophage activity than markers of CD68 and tumor necrosis factor-α, notably in coronary arteries.[68] This suggests [68Ga]DOTATATE could be a powerful tracer for detection of inflammation in arteries.[69] [68Ga]DOTATATE binding to CD68 macrophage-rich plaques has been validated by mRNA quantification.[70] Largely owing the promise of [68Ga]DOTATATE and related radiotracers for cardiovascular and cancer imaging, there is currently heavy demand for gallium-68 generators, which use the germanium-68 parent isotope. Although [68Ga]DOTATATE has been evaluated to detect atherosclerotic lesions, this tracer awaits further clinical studies to be established as a reliable inflammation imaging marker in coronary and carotid arteries in patients with CVD.[71]

[68Ga]Pentixafor

A recently developed PET radiotracer, [68Ga]pentixafor (see **Fig. 7**) binds with nanomolar affinity to C-X-C chemokine receptor type 4 (CXCR4), which is expressed on the outer membranes of inflammatory cells. This study used a rabbit model to detect the expression of CXCR4 in atherosclerotic plaques.[72,73] In addition to localizing in the liver

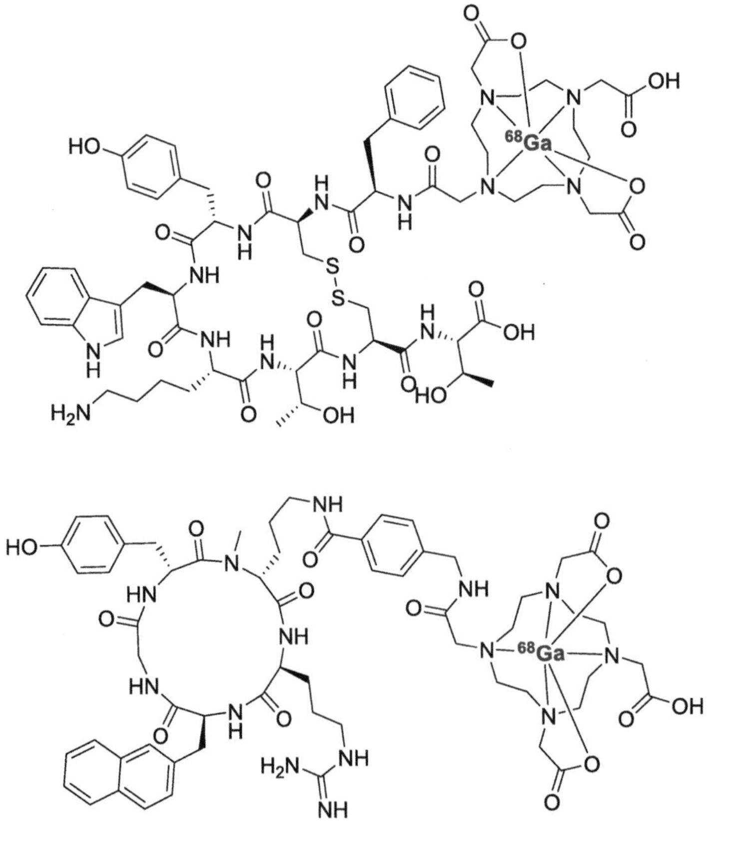

Fig. 7. Structures of [68Ga]DOTATATE (top) and [68Ga]pentixafor (bottom).

and kidneys, [⁶⁸Ga]pentixafor was detected in the right carotid arteries and abdominal aorta by PET imaging. Uptake was correlated with that of CXCR4 expression in the plaques, as detected by autoradiography.[73] In a clinical setting, [⁶⁸Ga]pentixafor was injected in patients with atherosclerosis and uptake was observed in human carotid atherosclerotic plaques. Therefore, [⁶⁸Ga]pentixafor represents a promising PET radiotracer useful in detecting CXCR4 expression on atherosclerotic plaques, and thereby directly determining the levels of macrophage infiltration in high risk plaques.[72]

[¹⁸F]FB-cAbVCAM-1–5 nanobody

By attracting monocytes and T lymphocytes to the developing lesions, vascular cell adhesion molecule-1 (VCAM-1) plays a crucial role in the progression of atherosclerosis.[74] After establishing clinically that single domain antibodies, also known as nanobodies, can be radiolabeled and safely administered to humans, many studies focused on using these antigen-binding 12-15 kDa fragments.[75] This study aimed to generate an anti–VCAM-1 ¹⁸F-labeled radiotracer ([¹⁸F]FB-cAbVCAM-1–5 Nb) for atherosclerosis imaging in apolipoprotein-E–deficient mice. Uptake in the excised aorta of mice with more advanced lesions were significantly higher than in mice with smaller lesions.[74] In addition, coinjection with 70-fold excess of unlabeled FB-cAbVCAM-1–5 Nb caused a significant decrease in aortic uptake, demonstrating tracer specificity. In addition to these results, the low myocardial uptake of [¹⁸F]FB-cAbVCAM-1–5 Nb makes it a promising tracer for atherosclerosis imaging in humans. However, further investigations are needed to assess the safety of [¹⁸F]FB-cAbVCAM-1–5 Nb in clinical trials.[75]

Matrix metalloproteinases

Matrix metalloproteinases (MMPs) are emerging as new targets for imaging lesion progression in atherosclerosis.[76] MMPs are Zn^{2+}-dependent endopeptidases and are responsible for remodeling of the extracellular matrix. Specifically, these proteins degrade collagen and may contribute to inflammation and destabilization of atherosclerotic lesions.[77] Radiolabeled MMP inhibitors are now the subject of numerous studies seeking to establish the importance of MMPs in inflammatory conditions.[78,79] Arguably the most advanced of these is the moderately selective gelatinase inhibitor [¹⁸F]BR351 (**Fig. 8**),[80] which has been deployed to detect remodeling after a stroke,[81,82] and whose analogs have been studied in the vasculature.[83] MMP imaging may be complicated by

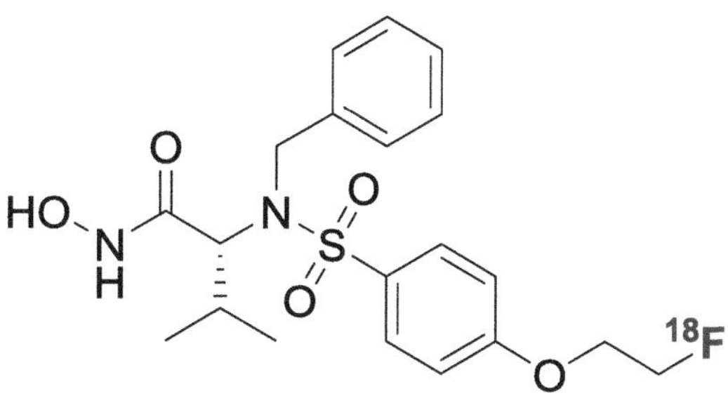

Fig. 8. Structure of [¹⁸F]BR351.

manifold isozymes with different biochemical substrates, expression levels in tissue, and pathologic roles. Therefore, highly sensitive and selective tracers are likely to be needed.

Fatty Acid Metabolism

The high metabolic rate of the heart makes it one of the most energy-consuming organs in the human body, with constant demands for ATP.[84] Mitochondrial oxidative phosphorylation is the main source for the continual production of ATP, followed by glycolysis and the tricarboxylic acid cycle. Fatty acid metabolism is an important contributor to meet myocardial demands for ATP; therefore, labeling components in the fatty acid pathway expands the understanding of fatty acid–related cardiovascular abnormalities, making it a clinically relevant pathway for imaging.[85] Shifts away from fatty acid metabolism can be a marker of pathology caused by different cardiomyopathic conditions, including ischemia and diabetes. Imaging fatty acid metabolic processes, therefore, leads to new insights into the mechanisms behind the development of myocardial pathology.[86]

[¹¹C]Acetate

Acetate is a salt that is readily taken up by cells to be activated by acetyl-coenzyme A (CoA) synthetase. Acetate is converted to acetyl-CoA in the mitochondria and cytosol.[87] In healthy myocardium, acetyl-CoA is metabolized to CO_2 through the TCA cycle.[88] Any abnormality in the CO_2 and acetate equilibrium affects the incorporation of cholesterol and fatty acids into cell membranes, leading to different cardiomyopathies.[88–90] [¹¹C]Acetate (**Fig. 9**) imaging is useful to observe overall oxidative metabolism in the myocardium. Changes can be indicative of the effects of acute ischemia, recovery of perfusion, and myocardial viability. [¹¹C]Acetate was also shown to be a better tracer to study MBF than [¹⁵O]water in patients with cardiomyopathy.[91] Heterogenous and reduced myocardial oxidative metabolic rate, cardiac efficiency, and output, as observed by [¹¹C]acetate imaging may suggest

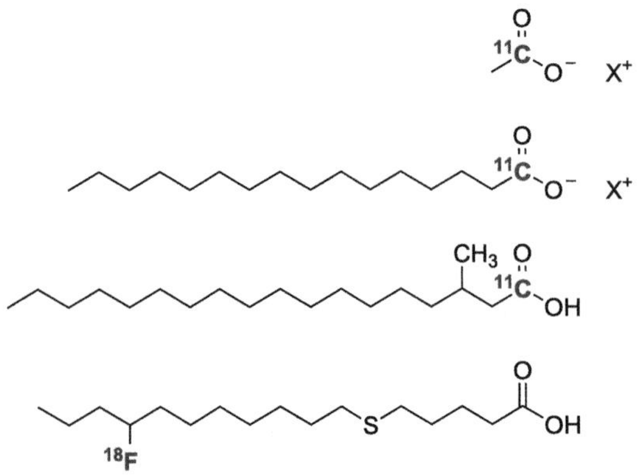

Fig. 9. Structures of [^{11}C]acetate, [^{11}C]palmitate, [^{11}C] BMHDA, and [^{18}F]FTHA.

cardiomyopathy.[92,93] [^{11}C]Acetate has also been studied to monitor vascular fatty acid metabolism in atherosclerosis. Although uptake does not closely match the distribution of calcified lesions, it has been suggested that this tracer could be useful to observe changes upon pharmacologic intervention.[94]

[^{11}C]Palmitate

The essential difference between [^{11}C]acetate and [^{11}C]palmitate (see **Fig. 9**) is that the latter is a long chain fatty acid, which can undergo oxidation, storage, redistribution, and clearance over the course of a PET scan.[95,96] Because long chain fatty acids make up the primary energy source for the myocardium, [^{11}C]palmitate uptake and clearance can provide insight into the pathophysiologic mechanisms in ischemic heart disease and cardiomyopathies. Although an advantage of [^{11}C]palmitate resides in the fact that it is indistinguishable from endogenous palmitate and shares a higher turnover rate, unfortunately, this property also results in complex kinetics that require metabolite correction and dynamic blood sampling for accurate image interpretation.[95]

[^{18}F]FTHA and [^{11}C]BMHDA

[^{18}F](R,S)-14-Fluoro-6-thia-heptadecanoic acid ([^{18}F]FTHA, see **Fig. 9**) is a radiolabeled long-chain fatty acid that acts similarly to [^{11}C]palmitate, but has a longer retention in the myocardium.[97] This observed metabolic trapping is due to the inhibited oxidation caused by 6-thia linkage in the fatty acid chain. DeGrado and colleagues[97] showed that [^{18}F]FTHA has high uptake in the rodent heart and its retention in the myocardium was suggested to be due to the tracer undergoing the initial metabolic steps in fatty acid oxidation. Therefore, the long chain or the sulfur atom do not hinder translocation of [^{18}F]FTHA to its binding

sites with albumin in the myocyte. In addition, metabolite analysis suggests that [^{18}F]FTHA is converted to its CoA adduct.[98–100] Similarly, [1-^{11}C]*beta*-methylheptadecanoic acid (BMHDA, see **Fig. 9**) was designed to prevent isotope liberation and clearance by impeding metabolic degradation.[101]

Cardiac Autonomic Nervous System

The autonomic nervous system supports cardiovascular homeostasis, metabolism, cardiac output, and vasoreactivity.[102] Faulty signaling in the autonomic nervous system owing to aging, stress, and cardiac events may contribute to the pathophysiology of heart failure, hypertension, and ischemic heart disease.[103] Norepinephrine is the main neurotransmitter in the sympathetic nervous system and stimulates increased force of contraction, conduction, and heart rate by the activation of β_1-adrenergic receptors.[102] Conversely, activation of cholinergic neurons in the parasympathetic nervous system by acetylcholine induces reduced cardiac activation through M_2 muscarinic receptors.[102]

[^{11}C]CGP12177

[^{11}C](S)-CGP12177 (**Fig. 10**) is a β_1/β_2 receptor antagonist and can be used to assess postsynaptic transmission.[102] [^{11}C]CGP12177 is currently the most well-characterized adrenergic receptor antagonist and is clinically used in PET to visualize β_1 and β_2 receptor density, which can aide in diagnosing patients with cardiomyopathies.[104] The production of [^{11}C](S)-CGP12177 currently relies on the use of [^{11}C]COCl$_2$ and 1-(3-*tert*-butylamino-2-hydroxypropoxy)-2,3-diamino benzene, can be synthesized with a molar activity of 0.54 to 1.08 Ci/μmol, and is suitable for human injection.[105] This tracer is still used in research, because it provides evidence for cardiac conditions such as heart failure and chronotropic incompetence, among other diseases that are symptomatic of adrenoceptor dysfunction.[104] Recently, cardiac PET was used to assess β-AR density in patients with chronotropic incompetence, and was shown to be downregulated.[104]

[^{11}C]MQNB

Quinuclidinyl benzilate (MQNB; see **Fig. 10**) is a M_1/M_2 antagonist with high specificity, and can be radiolabeled by reacting 3-quinuclinidyl benzilate with [^{11}C]MeI or [^{11}C]CH$_3$OTf, with decay corrected yields of 23%.[106,107] [^{11}C]MQNB can be used for imaging MR density for patients who have undergone heart transplantation, as well as those with chronic idiopathic dilated cardiomyopathy, familial amyloid neuropathy, myocardial infarctions, or congestive heart failure. It has been found that an upregulation of muscarinic receptors occurs in individuals with failing hearts.[27] Recently, this tracer has been used to image cardiac innervation in amyloidosis and is still used in the quantification of muscarinic receptor density.[108]

[^{11}C]Meta-hydroxyephedrine

The most clinically used PET radiotracer to study the sympathetic nervous system is [^{11}C]meta-hydroxyephedrine ([^{11}C]HED, see **Fig. 10**), a radiolabeled catecholamine analogue.[102] This tracer is known to bind to norepinephrine transporter, which is located in varicosities at the terminal axon and responsible for norepinephrine reuptake from the synaptic cleft.[103] [^{11}C]HED is synthesized by the N-methylation of metaraminol using [^{11}C]CH$_3$I, or [^{11}C]CH$_3$OTf, produced with a molar activity of greater than 370 GBq/μmol.[109] It is suggested that [^{11}C]HED is released continuously and recycled by the norepinephrine transporter in sympathetic neurons, because it shows high and sustained uptake over the course of a PET scan. [^{11}C]HED is currently used clinically to assess patients who have undergone heart transplantation, as well as those with suspected heart failure, cardiac diabetic neuropathy, and cardiomyopathy.[102] Interestingly, [^{11}C]HED has been used in conjunction with [^{11}C]CGP12177 to achieve complete assessment of sympathetic innervation for cardiac abnormalities.[109]

[^{18}F]LMI1195

Owing to the short half-life of ^{11}C, ^{18}F radiotracers with similar functions are increasingly sought after. [^{18}F]LMI1195 ([^{18}F]N-[3-bromo-4-(3-fluoro-propoxy)-benzyl]guanidine; see **Fig. 10**) shares structural features with the single-photon emitter [^{123}I]meta-iodobenzylguanidine ([^{123}I]MIBG) and

can also be used to assess cardiac sympathetic innervation.[110] [^{18}F]LMI1195 is synthesized from a brosylate precursor by a 1-step nucleophilic substitution reaction using [^{18}F]fluoride, and is obtained with greater than 95% radiochemical purity, with a specific activity of greater than 3.5 Ci/μmol.[111] The norepinephrine transporter inhibitor desipramine decreased [^{18}F]LMI1195 myocardial uptake by 82% with a maximum dose of 1 mg/kg, as shown by PET imaging in rabbits.[110] Direct tissue sampling (autoradiography) confirmed this finding.[110] Preliminary clinical findings with [^{18}F]LMI1195 have suggested it may provide more accurate measurements of cardiac sympathetic innervation in comparison with [^{11}C]HED, especially for early imaging.[112]

SUMMARY

Cardiovascular PET imaging is a powerful tool to evaluate markers of numerous CVDs, including atherosclerosis, ischemia, heart failure, and others, and relies on an armament of carefully refined radiopharmaceuticals probing an array of biochemical processes. Future PET radiopharmaceuticals for CVD are still needed, and will exploit new markers with greater mechanistic and disease specificity to advance diagnosis and clinical research.

REFERENCES

1. Mensah GA, Brown DW. An overview of cardiovascular disease burden in the United States. Health Aff (Millwood) 2007;26(1):38–48.
2. World Health Organization. The top 10 causes of death. Available at: http://www.who.int/news-room/fact-sheets/detail/the-top-10-causes-of-death. Accessed September 14, 2018.
3. Stewart J, Manmathan G, Wilkinson P. Primary prevention of cardiovascular disease: a review of

contemporary guidance and literature. JRSM Cardiovasc Dis 2017;6. 2048004016687211.

4. Cassar A, Holmes DR, Rihal CS, et al. Chronic coronary artery disease: diagnosis and management. Mayo Clin Proc 2009;84(12):1130–46.

5. Inamdar A, Inamdar A, Inamdar AA, et al. Heart failure: diagnosis, management and utilization. J Clin Med 2016;5(7):62.

6. Mozaffarian D, Benjamin EJ, Go AS, et al. Heart disease and stroke statistics–2015 update: a report from the American Heart Association. Circulation 2015;131(4):e29–322.

7. Blumgart HL, Weiss S. Studies on the velocity of blood flow. J Clin Invest 1927;4(3):399–425.

8. Prinzmetal M, Corday E, Bergman HC, et al. Radio-cardiography: a new method for studying the blood flow through the chambers of the heart in human beings. Science 1948;108(2804):340–1.

9. Slomka PJ, Dey D, Sitek A, et al. Cardiac imaging: working towards fully-automated machine analysis & interpretation. Expert Rev Med Devices 2017; 14(3):197–212.

10. Lameka K, Farwell MD, Ichise M. Positron emission tomography. Handb Clin Neurol 2016;135:209–27.

11. Li Y, Zhang W, Wu H, et al. Advanced tracers in PET imaging of cardiovascular disease. Biomed Res Int 2014;2014:1–13.

12. Conti M, Eriksson L. Physics of pure and non-pure positron emitters for PET: a review and a discussion. EJNMMI Phys 2016;3(1).

13. Coronary artery disease: overview. PubMed Health; 2017. Available at: https://www.ncbi.nlm.nih.gov/pubmedhealth/PMH0086334/. Accessed September 14, 2018.

14. Rischpler C, Park M-J, Fung GSK, et al. Advances in PET myocardial perfusion imaging: F-18 labeled tracers. Ann Nucl Med 2012;26(1):1–6.

15. Vedanthan R, Fuster V. The moving target of global cardiovascular health: disease prevention. Nat Rev Cardiol 2009;6(5):327–8.

16. Waldeck J, Molinos C, Gsell W, et al. Coincidence high-resolution and high-sensitivity PET imaging of cardiovascular disease: a powerful tool for disease imaging. Presented at: Bruker BioSpin MRI GmbH; December, 2017; Ettlingen, Germany. Available at: https://www.bruker.cn/fileadmin/user_upload/8-PDF-Docs/PreclinicalImaging/Concidence_High-Resolution_and_High-Sensitivity_PET_Imaging_of_Cardiovascular_Disease.pdf. Accessed September 13, 2018.

17. Chow BJW, Beanlands RS, Lee A, et al. Treadmill exercise produces larger perfusion defects than dipyridamole stress N-13 ammonia positron emission tomography. J Am Coll Cardiol 2006;47(2):411–6.

18. Bergmann SR, Hack S, Tewson T, et al. The dependence of accumulation of 13NH3 by myocardium on metabolic factors and its implications for quantitative assessment of perfusion. Circulation 1980;61(1):34–43.

19. Cheng KT. [13N]Ammonia. In: Molecular imaging and contrast agent database (MICAD). Bethesda (MD): National Center for Biotechnology Information (US); 2004. Available at: https://www.ncbi.nlm.nih.gov/pubmed/?term=20641280. Accessed September 15, 2018.

20. Bol A, Melin JA, Vanoverschelde JL, et al. Direct comparison of [13N]ammonia and [15O]water estimates of perfusion with quantification of regional myocardial blood flow by microspheres. Circulation 1993;87(2):512–25.

21. Nitzsche EU, Choi Y, Czernin J, et al. Noninvasive quantification of myocardial blood flow in humans. A direct comparison of the [13N]ammonia and the [15O]water techniques. Circulation 1996;93(11): 2000–6.

22. Cho S-G, Park KS, Kim J, et al. Coronary flow reserve and relative flow reserve measured by N-13 ammonia PET for characterization of coronary artery disease. Ann Nucl Med 2017;31(2):144–52.

23. Welch MJ, Kilbourn MR. A remote system for the routine production of oxygen-15 radiopharmaceuticals. J Labelled Comp Radiopharm 1985;22(11): 1193–200.

24. Renaud JM, Mylonas I, McArdle B, et al. Clinical interpretation standards and quality assurance for the multicenter PET/CT Trial rubidium-ARMI. J Nucl Med 2014;55(1):58–64.

25. Danad I, Raijmakers PG, Appelman YE, et al. Coronary risk factors and myocardial blood flow in patients evaluated for coronary artery disease: a quantitative [15O]H2O PET/CT study. Eur J Nucl Med Mol Imaging 2012;39(1):102–12.

26. Manabe O, Naya M, Aikawa T, et al. O-15-labeled water is the best myocardial blood flow tracer for precise MBF quantification. JNSC. http://doi.org/10.17996/anc.18-00064. 18-00064.

27. Dilsizian V, Taillefer R. Journey in evolution of nuclear cardiology. JACC Cardiovasc Imaging 2012; 5(12):1269–84.

28. Rubeaux M, Joshi NV, Dweck MR, et al. Motion correction of 18F-NaF PET for imaging coronary atherosclerotic plaques. J Nucl Med 2016;57(1): 54–9.

29. Berman DS, Maddahi J, Tamarappoo BK, et al. Flurpiridaz F 18 PET: phase II safety and clinical comparison with SPECT myocardial perfusion imaging for detection of coronary artery disease. J Am Coll Cardiol 2013;61(4):469–77.

30. Maddahi J, Czernin J, Berman D, et al. Comparison of flurpiridaz F 18 PET injection and Tc-99m labeled SPECT myocardial perfusion imaging for identifying severity and extent of stress induced myocardial ischemia in phase 2 clinical trials. J Nucl Med 2011;52(supplement 1):444.

31. Love WD, Romney RB, Burch GE. A comparison of the distribution of potassium and exchangeable rubidium in the organs of the dog, using rubidium [86]. Circ Res 1954;2(2):112–22.

32. Huang SC, Williams BA, Krivokapich J, et al. Rabbit myocardial 82Rb kinetics and a compartmental model for blood flow estimation. Am J Physiol 1989;256(4):H1156–64.

33. Herrero P, Markham J, Shelton ME, et al. Noninvasive quantification of regional myocardial perfusion with rubidium-82 and positron emission tomography. Exploration of a mathematical model. Circulation 1990;82(4):1377–86.

34. Hsu B. PET tracers and techniques for measuring myocardial blood flow in patients with coronary artery disease. J Biomed Res 2013;27(6):452–9.

35. Selwyn AP, Allan RM, L'Abbate A, et al. Relation between regional myocardial uptake of rubidium-82 and perfusion: absolute reduction of cation uptake in ischemia. Am J Cardiol 1982;50(1):112–21.

36. Chatal J-F, Rouzet F, Haddad F, et al. Story of rubidium-82 and advantages for myocardial perfusion PET imaging. Front Med (Lausanne) 2015;2.

37. Posani K, Menda Y, Graham M, et al. Head to head comparison of N-13 ammonia and Rubidium-82 PET myocardial perfusion scans in subjects with no history of coronary artery disease (CAD). J Nucl Med 2012;53(supplement 1):1816.

38. Gurm GS, Danik SB, Shoup TM, et al. 4-[18F]-tetraphenylphosphonium as a PET tracer for myocardial mitochondrial membrane potential. JACC Cardiovasc Imaging 2012;5(3):285–92.

39. Kadenbach B, Ramzan R, Moosdorf R, et al. The role of mitochondrial membrane potential in ischemic heart failure. Mitochondrion 2011;11(5):700–6.

40. Zielonka J, Joseph J, Sikora A, et al. Mitochondria-targeted triphenylphosphonium-based compounds: syntheses, mechanisms of action, and therapeutic and diagnostic applications. Chem Rev 2017;117(15):10043–120.

41. Lusis AJ. Atherosclerosis. Nature 2000;407:233.

42. Suzuki H, Kurihara Y, Takeya M, et al. A role for macrophage scavenger receptors in atherosclerosis and susceptibility to infection. Nature 1997;386(6622):292–6.

43. Rodondi N, Marques-Vidal P, Butler J, et al. Markers of atherosclerosis and inflammation for prediction of coronary heart disease in older adults. Am J Epidemiol 2010;171(5):540–9.

44. Cocker MS, Spence JD, Hammond R, et al. [18F]-fluorodeoxyglucose PET/CT imaging as a marker of carotid plaque inflammation: comparison to immunohistology and relationship to acuity of events. Int J Cardiol 2018;271:378–86.

45. Wakabayashi H, Werner R, Hayakawa N, et al. Focal 18F-FDG uptake in acute inflammation is associated with CD68-positive macrophage infiltration in a rat model of autoimmune myocarditis. J Nucl Med 2016;57(supplement 2):395.

46. Bhambhvani P. Challenges of cardiac inflammation imaging with F-18 FDG positron emission tomography. J Nucl Cardiol 2017;24(1):100–2.

47. Gigengack F, Ruthotto L, Burger M, et al. Motion correction in dual gated cardiac PET using mass-preserving image registration. IEEE Trans Med Imaging 2012;31(3):698–712.

48. Vengrenyuk Y, Carlier S, Xanthos S, et al. A hypothesis for vulnerable plaque rupture due to stress-induced debonding around cellular microcalcifications in thin fibrous caps. Proc Natl Acad Sci U S A 2006;103(40):14678–83.

49. Blau M, Ganatra R, Bender MA. 18 F-fluoride for bone imaging. Semin Nucl Med 1972;2(1):31–7.

50. Pell VR, Baark F, Mota F, et al. PET imaging of cardiac hypoxia: hitting hypoxia where it hurts. Curr Cardiovasc Imaging Rep 2018;11(3).

51. Tarkin JM, Joshi FR, Rudd JHF. PET imaging of inflammation in atherosclerosis. Nat Rev Cardiol 2014;11(8):443–57.

52. Joshi FR, Manavaki R, Fryer TD, et al. Vascular Imaging with 18F-fluorodeoxyglucose positron emission tomography is influenced by hypoxia. J Am Coll Cardiol 2017;69(14):1873–4.

53. Folco EJ, Sheikine Y, Rocha VZ, et al. Hypoxia but not inflammation augments glucose uptake in human macrophages: implications for imaging atherosclerosis with 18fluorine-labeled 2-deoxy-D-glucose positron emission tomography. J Am Coll Cardiol 2011;58(6):603–14.

54. Krohn KA, Link JM, Mason RP. Molecular imaging of hypoxia. J Nucl Med 2008;49(Suppl 2):129S–48S.

55. Mateo J, Izquierdo-Garcia D, Badimon JJ, et al. Noninvasive assessment of hypoxia in rabbit advanced atherosclerosis using 18F-fluoromisonidazole PET imaging. Circ Cardiovasc Imaging 2014;7(2):312–20.

56. van der Valk FM, Sluimer JC, Voo SA, et al. In vivo imaging of hypoxia in atherosclerotic plaques in humans. JACC Cardiovasc Imaging 2015;8(11):1340–1.

57. Nie X, Randolph GJ, Elvington A, et al. Imaging of hypoxia in mouse atherosclerotic plaques with ^{64}Cu-ATSM. Nucl Med Biol 2016;43(9):534–42.

58. Nie X, Laforest R, Elvington A, et al. PET/MRI of hypoxic atherosclerosis using 64Cu-ATSM in a rabbit model. J Nucl Med 2016;57(12):2006–11.

59. Medina RA, Mariotti E, Pavlovic D, et al. 64Cu-CTS: a promising radiopharmaceutical for the identification of low-grade cardiac hypoxia by PET. J Nucl Med 2015;56(6):921–6.

60. Cumming P, Burgher B, Patkar O, et al. Sifting through the surfeit of neuroinflammation tracers. J Cereb Blood Flow Metab 2018;38(2):204–22.

61. Fujimura Y, Hwang PM, Trout H III, et al. Increased peripheral benzodiazepine receptors in arterial plaque of patients with atherosclerosis: an autoradiographic study with [3H]PK 11195. Atherosclerosis 2008;201(1):108–11.

62. Pugliese F, Gaemperli O, Kinderlerer AR, et al. Imaging of vascular inflammation with [11C]-PK11195 and positron emission tomography/computed tomography angiography. J Am Coll Cardiol 2010; 56(8):653–61.

63. Laitinen I, Saraste A, Weidl E, et al. Evaluation of v 3 integrin-targeted positron emission tomography tracer 18F-Galacto-RGD for imaging of vascular inflammation in atherosclerotic mice. Circ Cardiovasc Imaging 2009;2(4):331–8.

64. Gaemperli O, Shalhoub J, Owen DRJ, et al. Imaging intraplaque inflammation in carotid atherosclerosis with 11C-PK11195 positron emission tomography/computed tomography. Eur Heart J 2012;33(15):1902–10.

65. Thackeray JT, Hupe HC, Wang Y, et al. Myocardial inflammation predicts remodeling and neuroinflammation after myocardial infarction. J Am Coll Cardiol 2018;71(3):263–75.

66. Notni J, Steiger K, Hoffmann F, et al. Complementary, selective PET imaging of integrin subtypes α5β1 and αvβ3 using 68Ga-aquibeprin and 68Ga-avebetrin. J Nucl Med 2016;57(3):460–6.

67. Tarkin JM, Joshi FR, Evans NR, et al. Detection of atherosclerotic inflammation by 68Ga-DOTATATE PET compared to [18F]FDG PET imaging. J Am Coll Cardiol 2017;69(14):1774–91.

68. Pedersen SF, Sandholt BV, Keller SH, et al. 64Cu-DOTATATE PET/MRI for detection of activated macrophages in carotid atherosclerotic plaques. Arterioscler Thromb Vasc Biol 2015;35(7):1696–703.

69. Reubi JC, Schär J-C, Waser B, et al. Affinity profiles for human somatostatin receptor subtypes SST1–SST5 of somatostatin radiotracers selected for scintigraphic and radiotherapeutic use. Eur J Nucl Med 2000;27(3):273–82.

70. Joshi NV, Vesey AT, Williams MC, et al. 18F-fluoride positron emission tomography for identification of ruptured and high-risk coronary atherosclerotic plaques: a prospective clinical trial. Lancet 2014; 383(9918):705–13.

71. Schatka I, Wollenweber T, Haense C, et al. Peptide receptor–targeted radionuclide therapy alters inflammation in atherosclerotic plaques. J Am Coll Cardiol 2013;62(24):2344–5.

72. Hyafil F, Pelisek J, Laitinen I, et al. Imaging the cytokine receptor CXCR4 in atherosclerotic plaques with the radiotracer 68Ga-Pentixafor for PET. J Nucl Med 2017;58(3):499–506.

73. Hyafil F, Cornily J-C, Rudd JHF, et al. Quantification of inflammation within rabbit atherosclerotic plaques using the macrophage-specific CT contrast agent N1177: a comparison with 18F-FDG PET/CT and histology. J Nucl Med 2009; 50(6):959–65.

74. Nahrendorf M, McCarthy JR, Libby P. Over a hump for imaging atherosclerosis. Circ Res 2012;110(7): 902–3. Available at: https://www.ahajournals.org/doi/full/10.1161/CIRCRESAHA.112.267260. Accessed September 14, 2018.

75. Broisat A, Hernot S, Toczek J, et al. Nanobodies targeting mouse/human VCAM1 for the nuclear imaging of atherosclerotic lesions. Circ Res 2012;110(7): 927–37.

76. Visse R, Nagase H. Matrix metalloproteinases and tissue inhibitors of metalloproteinases: structure, function, and biochemistry. Circ Res 2003;92(8): 827–39.

77. Roycik MD, Myers JS, Newcomer RG, et al. Matrix metalloproteinase inhibition in atherosclerosis and stroke. Curr Mol Med 2013;13(8):1299–313.

78. Hugenberg V, Hermann S, Galla F, et al. Radiolabeled hydroxamate-based matrix metalloproteinase inhibitors: how chemical modifications affect pharmacokinetics and metabolic stability. Nucl Med Biol 2016;43(7):424–37.

79. Newby AC. Metalloproteinases promote plaque rupture and myocardial infarction: a persuasive concept waiting for clinical translation. Matrix Biol 2015;44-46:157–66.

80. Wagner S, Faust A, Breyholz H-J, et al. The MMP inhibitor (R)-2-(N-benzyl-4-(2-[18F]fluoroethoxy) phenylsulphonamido)-N-hydroxy-3-methylbutanamide: improved precursor synthesis and fully automated radiosynthesis. Appl Radiat Isot 2011;69(6): 862–8.

81. Zinnhardt B, Viel T, Wachsmuth L, et al. Multimodal imaging reveals temporal and spatial microglia and matrix metalloproteinase activity after experimental stroke. J Cereb Blood Flow Metab 2015;35(11): 1711–21.

82. Gerwien H, Hermann S, Zhang X, et al. Imaging matrix metalloproteinase activity in multiple sclerosis as a specific marker of leukocyte penetration of the blood-brain barrier. Sci Transl Med 2016; 8(364):364ra152.

83. Schäfers M, Riemann B, Kopka K, et al. Scintigraphic imaging of matrix metalloproteinase activity in the arterial wall in vivo. Circulation 2004; 109(21):2554–9.

84. Lopaschuk GD, Ussher JR, Folmes CDL, et al. Myocardial fatty acid metabolism in health and disease. Physiol Rev 2010;90(1):207–58.

85. Neely JR, Morgan HE. Relationship between carbohydrate and lipid metabolism and the energy balance of heart muscle. Annu Rev Physiol 1974; 36(1):413–59.

86. Giedd KN, Bergmann SR. Fatty acid imaging of the heart. Curr Cardiol Rep 2011;13(2):121–31.

87. Leung K. [11C]Acetate. In: Molecular imaging and contrast agent database (MICAD). Bethesda (MD): National Center for Biotechnology Information (US); 2004. Available at: https://www.ncbi.nlm.nih.gov/pubmed/?term=20641536. Accessed September 15, 2018.

88. Howard BV, Howard WJ. Lipids in normal and tumor cells in culture. Prog Biochem Pharmacol 1975;10:135–66.

89. Swinnen JV, Heemers H, Deboel L, et al. Stimulation of tumor-associated fatty acid synthase expression by growth factor activation of the sterol regulatory element-binding protein pathway. Oncogene 2000;19(45):5173–81.

90. Blaise G, Noël J, Vinay P, et al. Metabolic effects of acetate on the heart. Clin Invest Med 1989;12(4): 254–61.

91. Timmer SAJ, Lubberink M, Germans T, et al. Potential of [11C]acetate for measuring myocardial blood flow: studies in normal subjects and patients with hypertrophic cardiomyopathy. J Nucl Cardiol 2010;17(2):264–75.

92. Naya M, Tamaki N. Imaging of myocardial oxidative metabolism in heart failure. Curr Cardiovasc Imaging Rep 2014;7(1).

93. Grassi I, Nanni C, Allegri V, et al. The clinical use of PET with 11C-acetate. Am J Nucl Med Mol Imaging 2011;2(1):33–47.

94. Derlin T, Habermann CR, Lengyel Z, et al. Feasibility of 11C-Acetate PET/CT for imaging of fatty acid synthesis in the atherosclerotic vessel wall. J Nucl Med 2011;52(12):1848–54.

95. Christensen NL, Jakobsen S, Schacht AC, et al. Whole-body biodistribution, dosimetry, and metabolite correction of [11C]Palmitate: a PET tracer for imaging of fatty acid metabolism. Mol Imaging 2017; 16. https://doi.org/10.1177/1536012117734485.

96. Gupta S, Knight AG, Gupta S, et al. Saturated long chain fatty acids activate inflammatory signaling in astrocytes. J Neurochem 2012;120(6):1060–71.

97. DeGrado TR, Coenen HH, Stocklin G. 14(R,S)-[Fluoro-6-Thia-Heptadecanoic Acid (FTHA): Evaluation in Mouse of a New Probe of Myocardial Utilization of Long Chain Fatty Acids. J Nucl Med 1991;32: 1888–96.

98. Shoup TM, Elmaleh DR, Bonab AA, et al. Evaluation of trans-9-18F-fluoro-3,4-Methyleneheptadecanoic acid as a PET tracer for myocardial fatty acid imaging. J Nucl Med 2005;46(2):297–304.

99. Mather KJ, DeGrado T. Imaging of myocardial fatty acid oxidation. Biochim Biophys Acta 2016; 1860(10):1535–43.

100. Sankaralingam S, Lopaschuk GD. Cardiac energy metabolic alterations in pressure overload-

induced left and right heart failure (2013 Grover Conference Series). Pulm Circ 2015;5(1):15–28.

101. Pandey MK, Bansal A, DeGrado TR. Fluorine-18 labeled thia fatty acids for PET imaging of fatty acid oxidation in heart and cancer. Heart Metab 2011;(51):15–9.

102. Langer O, Halldin C. PET and SPET tracers for mapping the cardiac nervous system. Eur J Nucl Med 2002;29(3):416–34.

103. Shu Z, Zhu X. The widely used SPECT and PET tracers for cardiac sympathetic nervous system. Nucl Med Biomed Imaging 2017;2(3).

104. Goto T, Kikuchi S, Mori K, et al. Abstract 17070: impact of cardiac beta-adrenergic receptor density evaluated by cardiac PET on chronotropic incompetence. Circulation 2017. Available at: https://www.ahajournals.org/doi/abs/10.1161/circ.136.suppl_1.17070. Accessed September 14, 2018.

105. Boullais C, Crouzel C, Syrota A. Synthesis of 4-(3-t-butylamino-2-hydroxypropoxy)-benzimidazol-2(11c)-one (cgp 12177). J Labelled Comp Radiopharm 1986;23(5):565–7.

106. Dollé F, Hinnen F, Vaufrey F, et al. Highly efficient synthesis of [11C]Me-QNB, a selective radioligand for the quantification of the cardiac muscarinic receptors using PET. J Labelled Comp Radiopharm 2001;44:337–45.

107. Maziere M, Berger G, Godot J-M, et al. 11C-methiodide quinuclidinyl benzilate a muscarinic antagonist for in vivo studies of myocardial muscarinic receptors. J Radioanal Chem 1983;76(2):305–9.

108. Slart RHJA, Glaudemans AWJM, Hazenberg BPC, et al. Imaging cardiac innervation in amyloidosis. J Nucl Cardiol 2017. https://doi.org/10.1007/s12350-017-1059-9.

109. Shao X, Hoareau R, Runkle AC, et al. Highlighting the versatility of the Tracerlab synthesis modules. Part 2: fully automated production of [11C]-labeled radiopharmaceuticals using a Tracerlab FXC-Pro: production of [11C] radiopharmaceuticals using a Tracerlab FXC-Pro. J Labelled Comp Radiopharm 2011;54(14):819–38.

110. Yu M, Bozek J, Lamoy M, et al. Evaluation of LMI1195, a novel 18F-labeled cardiac neuronal pet imaging agent, in cells and animal models. Circ Cardiovasc Imaging 2011;4(4):435–43.

111. Noordzij W, Slart RHJA. PET imaging of the autonomic myocardial function: methods and interpretation. Clin Transl Imaging 2015;3(5):365–72.

112. Zelt J, Renaud J, Mielniczuk L, et al. Fluorine-18 Lmi1195 positron emission tomography provides accurate measure of cardiac sympathetic innervation compared to carbon-11 hydroxyephedrine. J Am Coll Cardiol 2018;71(11 Supplement):A1482.

Moving?

Make sure your subscription moves with you!

To notify us of your new address, find your **Clinics Account Number** (located on your mailing label above your name), and contact customer service at:

Email: journalscustomerservice-usa@elsevier.com

800-654-2452 (subscribers in the U.S. & Canada)
314-447-8871 (subscribers outside of the U.S. & Canada)

Fax number: 314-447-8029

Elsevier Health Sciences Division
Subscription Customer Service
3251 Riverport Lane
Maryland Heights, MO 63043

*To ensure uninterrupted delivery of your subscription, please notify us at least 4 weeks in advance of move.